AIDS and HIV

The nursing response

Edited by

Jean Faugier and Ian Hicken

North West Regional Health Authority
and School of Nursing Studies,
University of Manchester,
UK

CHAPMAN & HALL

London · Glasgow · Weinheim · New York · Tokyo · Melbourne · Madras

Published by Chapman & Hall, 2–6 Boundary Row, London SE1 8HN, UK

Chapman & Hall, 2–6 Boundary Row, London SE1 8HN, UK

Blackie Academic & Professional, Wester Cleddens Road, Bishopbriggs, Glasgow G64 2NZ, UK

Chapman & Hall GmbH, Pappelallee 3, 69469 Weinheim, Germany

Chapman & Hall USA, 115 Fifth Avenue, New York, NY 10003, USA

Chapman & Hall Japan, ITP-Japan, Kyowa Building, 3F, 2-2-1 Hirakawacho, Chiyoda-ku, Tokyo 102, Japan

Chapman & Hall Australia, 102 Dodds Street, South Melbourne, Victoria 3205, Australia

Chapman & Hall India, R. Seshadri, 32 Second Main Road, CIT East, Madras 600 035, India

Distributed in the USA and Canada by Singular Publishing Group Inc., 4284 41st Street, San Diego, California 92105

First edition 1996

Typeset in 8/9.5 pt. Times by Saxon Graphics Ltd, Derby
Printed in Great Britain by Hartnolls Ltd, Bodmin, Cornwall

ISBN 0 412 56090 9   1 56593 585 3 (USA)

A catalogue record for this book is available from the British Library

Library of Congress Catalog Card Number: 95-74662

This book is dedicated to the memory of Richard Wells

Contents

Contributors

Neil Brocklehurst
Primary Care Development
    Researcher
Sandwell Family Health Services
    Authority
West Midlands
UK

Carmel Clancy
Research Fellow
St George's Hospital Medical
    School
London
UK

Patrick Coyne
Clinical Nurse Specialist/Honorary
    Research Associate
Riverside Mental Health Trust
Substance Misuse Services
London
UK

Steve Cranfield
Independent Trainer and
    Researcher
London
UK

Jean Faugier
Regional Director of Nursing
North West Regional Health
Authority

and Senior Lecturer
School of Nursing Studies
University of Manchester
UK

Steven Firn
Lecturer/Practitioner in HIV and
    Mental Health
The Bethlem Royal Hospital
London
UK

Tony Harrison
Nurse Tutor
Manchester College of Midwifery
    and Nursing
Ashton under Lyne
UK

Mavis Hibbard
Family Services Manager
The Mildmay Mission Hospital
London
UK
(until March, 1995)

Ian Hicken
Research Fellow
Community Nursing Professorial
    Unit
University of Manchester
UK

Sarah Holmes-Smith
Locality Manager
Community Mental Health Team
City and Hackney NHS Trust
London
UK

John Hooker
Senior Nurse (Commissioning)
South of Tyne Health Commission
UK

Carol Pellowe
Assistant Director
Centre for Sexual Health and HIV
    Studies
Thames Valley University
London
UK

Geraldine Reilly
Clinical Nurse Specialist
Chelsea and Westminster Hospital

London
UK

Carol Smith
Senior Liaison Nurse (HIV)
Central Middlesex Hospital
London
UK

Margaret A. Worsley
Senior Nurse Manager
North Manchester General
    Hospital
UK

Steve Wright
Director
TENDA
Camden House
Ashton under Lyne
UK

Foreword

After being involved in work associated with nursing and HIV infection since 1985, I was greatly honoured to be invited to write the foreword to this book.

Since the early to mid-1980s, when the AIDS pandemic took hold in this country, there has been a wide variety of responses from health and social care authorities. Indeed, the thirst for knowledge in the subject transcends much of what is already known about other sexually transmitted or infectious diseases. It is therefore essential for us to harness these responses in order to ensure that the broadest spectrum of care required by individuals with HIV infection is delivered in a measured and coordinated way.

As a nursing officer at government level prior to my retirement, I was in the fortunate position of being able to see how some of these responses were initiated, carried forward and brought to fruition. Through my personal contact with the co-editors of this book, I have witnessed at first-hand their commitment to the totality of care, which includes diagnostic, clinical, continuing, pastoral and psychological dimensions: it is therefore without any reservation that I now promote this book to wide attention.

The individual writers bring an extensive knowledge of AIDS and HIV-related diseases, each chapter adding its own specialist contribution to what can only be described as a comprehensive picture of the overall needs of patients/clients and their friends and relatives, as well as an in-depth analysis of the best health-care provision that can be offered by nurses, midwives or health visitors.

As we are all aware, the goalposts in HIV disease are forever moving, and the professions have to be adaptable and motivated to move with them. Many colleagues who are sadly no longer with us have pioneered the way, and the publication of this book enables the process of care which they identified to continue. It is my fervent hope that the book will be required reading and available in the widest possible arena.

Tom Snee OBE
HIV/Sexual Health Consultant
Surrey
UK

Acknowledgements

The editors would like to thank the following people for their help and support during the development of this book: Eileen Rendall, secretary at the Community Nursing Professorial Unit; Régis Faugier and Luis Casas.

PART ONE
Developing the Professional Infrastructure

INTRODUCTION

AIDS and HIV disease is the most devastating personal and public health problem we have faced this century. This book developed from the need to examine our response as a profession to the challenges posed by a problem of such enormous and all-encompassing proportions. This is not a 'textbook' to tell you all about the disease and its consequences for the individual who becomes infected. It will not deal with issues of biology, epidemiology or transmission in any detail. It is our view that all these issues have been and continue to be covered effectively in other books by writers with much more in-depth knowledge than ourselves or our contributors.

What this book is about is attempting to draw together lessons from the nursing response to the first decade of the pandemic in the UK. Since the early 1980s there have been impressive scientific advances in understanding of the AIDS virus, its transmission routes and its biological mechanisms. Although progress must seem painfully slow to those outside the field and even more tortuous to those with the disease, great strides have been made. However, these hard-won discoveries and breakthroughs have not led to the discovery of the 'cure' or the 'vaccine' that will make redundant the need for prevention or care. It is now accepted that the road to a vaccine will be long and arduous, involving quite mind-boggling commitments economically and enormous cooperative research efforts.

In the meantime the only way to prevent the spread of HIV is through education and other public health measures. And while the treatment regimens for those with AIDS are improving all the time and have resulted in increased life expectancy and improved quality of life, it remains the case that what really matters ultimately is the quality of support and care that people – many of them very young – receive in dealing with what remains a fatal disease.

The challenge of providing such care falls to nurses more often than to any other group of professionals, and while no one would suggest that everything in the garden is rosy there is much of which to be proud in the response of the profession to HIV and AIDS.

The chapters in this first section set out essential professional messages in order that we should get the 'infrastructure' right before we embark on anything else. Fundamental issues of strategic planning, ethical dilemmas, supervision and support and the contribution of research and education initiatives are explored fully by authors who are expert practitioners in these fields. Numerous examples are provided of how nurses are meeting the challenges posed by HIV and AIDS. Any new condition with the potential of HIV is bound by its very nature to expose a wide range of controversial dilemmas and contested approaches. Approaches to HIV testing, counselling and partner notification, educational needs and the question of attitudes to sensitive topics, the use of research findings and the provision of supervision and support, have all in their own way caused problems for those involved in HIV/AIDS nursing and no doubt will continue to do so.

All too often services wishing to provide a response to particular health needs in the community do so without giving due consideration as to how these issues should be organized to support and inform that response. The chapters in this section will, it is anticipated, go some way to informing the debate on these issues and shaping the response of nurses over the next decade.

In addition, it is important to recognize that it is not only nursing that needs to give consideration to these fundamental professional issues. They are, and should be, of concern to many other branches of the medical profession, and the experience in HIV and AIDS can provide important lessons for all nurses in today's uncertain world.

Strategic planning in the era of AIDS

1

Ian Hicken and Jean Faugier

INTRODUCTION

'HIV and AIDS has secured its place as one of the significant and sinister medical puzzles of this or any other generation. It has also achieved eminence as providing some of the most compelling examples of interaction between biomedical and psychosocial variables' (Cawley, 1988).

Nurses throughout the world have responded admirably to the challenges posed by this complex and multifarious disease. Innovative nursing practices, informed by research, intuition, consultation and collaboration, have been developed and implemented in an attempt to alleviate and minimize the personal and social impact of HIV infection. The nursing profession has responded to HIV within an established framework of health and social policy which has influenced and shaped models of professional practice.

Some years before the emergence of HIV, in 1978, in the Declaration of Alma Ata, the World Health Organization (WHO) issued a challenge to the countries of the world to attain 'health for all by the year 2000' (WHO, 1978). This included six major themes which were to have a direct impact on the future of HIV-related medical and nursing practice, with a shift in focus to health promotion and disease prevention, involving community participation and multisectorial cooperation. The issue of equity in health care was also seen as crucial, and primary health care as fundamental in providing readily accessible services as close as possible to where people live and work, with full community participation (WHO, 1985). At a broader level, international cooperation has now become a key theme in recognition that some health problems transcend national frontiers.

In the 1980s, as knowledge and awareness about HIV infection grew and matured, it became increasingly evident that the framework for 'health for all by the year 2000' issued by WHO was an ideal flawed by political and social unrest, social injustice and discrimination, poverty and starvation, homelessness and unemployment, and inadequate resources. HIV and AIDS was, in part, responsible for highlighting the deficiencies in the prerequisites for health for all. Strategic planning for HIV and AIDS aimed to provide a framework for health and social care professionals within which they could respond to the needs of communities and individuals. Nurses have been at the forefront of that response, providing information, delivering HIV-related services and working in close collaboration with other health and social care professionals and non-governmental organizations.

This chapter aims to provide an overview of the global AIDS strategy and the United Kingdom response. It concludes by exploring how nurses have risen to the challenge of HIV and AIDS, and proposes that, on a professional and personal level, nurses still have much to do if they are to effectively meet the needs of HIV and non-HIV infected patients and clients.

THE GLOBAL RESPONSE

The World Health Organization (WHO) has been at the forefront of orchestrating and coordinating the health profession's response to HIV/AIDS in over 180 countries around the world. As a specialized agency of the United Nations, WHO has a primary responsibility for international health matters. Explicit in this responsibility is a role in coordinating the global strategy for the prevention and control of AIDS. Originally developed in 1985–86, the global AIDS strategy set out a framework for action which aimed to prevent infection with HIV, reduce the personal and social impact of HIV infection and mobilize and unify national and international efforts against AIDS (WHO, 1986).

In 1992, WHO published an update of the global AIDS strategy which brought together 'technically and ethically sound approaches of known effectiveness for meeting the pandemic's new challenges' (Merson, 1992). Informed by various scientific advances and a range of 'tried and tested' practical interventions, the 1992 global AIDS strategy provides a useful yet ideological framework for health professionals, governments and individuals to formulate responses to HIV/AIDS.

Although the main objectives of the strategy remain as relevant today as they were in 1986, new priorities in the evolving pandemic have been identified:

- an increased emphasis on the adequate and equitable provision of health care;
- expanded and more effective treatment for other sexually transmitted diseases;
- a reduction of the special vulnerability to HIV infection of women and their offspring;
- the creation of a more supportive social environment for AIDS prevention;
- immediate planning in anticipation of the socioeconomic impact of the pandemic;
- a greater focus on communicating effectively the compelling public health rationale for overcoming stigmatization and discrimination.

(WHO, 1992)

The global AIDS strategy is not without its critics, who questioned the efficacy of global strategies in relation to AIDS. According to Decosas (1993): 'To try to extrapolate from the responses of homosexual groups in metropolitan North America a strategy for AIDS throughout the world was a 'scandalous' error'. Decosas advocated instead tailor-made local responses, in harmony with the special mores and different attitudes of each distinct society, adding that increased global spending on AIDS was not the answer. What Decosas appears to have overlooked in adopting this standpoint is that, for many nations and societies around the world, AIDS is in danger of paling into insignificance given the many pressing social and political agendas that require urgent attention. Without a global AIDS strategy, those less empowered, socially and politically, are left without direction and solidarity. Perhaps one benefit of such a strategy is that it has given credence to the efforts of HIV/AIDS pioneers in their attempts to develop national AIDS programmes.

NATIONAL AIDS PROGRAMMES

Since the emergence and acknowledgement of HIV in the early 1980s, many nations have developed and established national AIDS programmes in an attempt to minimize the further spread of the virus. The Global AIDS Policy Coalition (1993) suggested that initially, early efforts to influence behaviour were solely dependent on the provision of information about safer behaviour and the dangers of AIDS. However, it soon became evident that information alone was not sufficient to achieve behavioural change. The evolutionary response to AIDS saw the emergence, within communities, of a mix of information, materials and services designed to promote behavioural change in specific groups of people, i.e. a programme-based approach responding to the identified needs of specific communities. The lessons learnt from this kind of approach were adopted on a wider scale by some countries and articulated by WHO in the shape of the first global AIDS strategy (Global AIDS Policy Coalition, 1993). Since the mid-1980s, strategic planning for HIV/AIDS has focused on the adaptation of a global model to local and national circumstances.

The global AIDS strategy and national AIDS programmes have without doubt helped focus our efforts against the HIV/AIDS pandemic but, despite those efforts, HIV infection continues to increase in all populations of the world (Merson, 1994). In an address to the 1993 Conference of European Community Parliamentarians on HIV/AIDS, Mann (1993) stated that 'the epidemic is still doing better against us than we are doing against it'. Similarly, in his address to delegates attending the 10th International Conference on AIDS in Japan, Merson (1994) posed a simple but poignant question: 'Why, if we know so much about preventing AIDS, is the epidemic continuing to expand?' He went on to say that, globally, over 6000 people are becoming infected with HIV every day and that 'the answers to the challenges of HIV depend on researchers, government officials, clinicians, journalists, citizens of all nations, men and women living with and without AIDS'. He called for greater unification from all concerned and stressed the need for all possible allies 'to seek each other out and link up'. Could it be that, despite a 'corporate' voice about the issues, there remains widespread disparity as to how best to learn from and capitalize on our experiences?

Over recent years it has become evident that national AIDS programmes and the global AIDS strategy have their limitations. Several reasons have been put forward to explain why, despite intensive action, the level of behavioural change has been insufficient to halt or substantially slow the spread of HIV (Global AIDS Policy Coalition, 1993). Poor communication, inadequate mechanisms for disseminating examples of good practice, isolation of HIV/AIDS work from other health programmes and activities, a fading sense of purpose and direction, difficulty in identifying and responding to the needs of diverse populations, and increasing bureaucracy, have all been cited as contributing factors. Clearly, there appears to be a consensus of opinion that international and national efforts are not achieving the desired goals of preventing infection with HIV; reducing the personal and social impact of HIV infection; mobilizing and unifying national and international efforts against AIDS. However, it is possible to speculate that, without a common global agenda for HIV/AIDS, we would be seeing infection rates escalating at a greater rate than current monitoring and surveillance suggests.

A NEW FOCUS FOR AN AIDS STRATEGY?

Work to date on HIV and AIDS programme-based strategies has shown that prevention efforts can succeed if they include three basic elements, i.e. information and education, health and social services and a supportive environment – the 'prevention triad' (Global AIDS Policy Coalition, 1993). However, increasing evidence would suggest that there is a critical relationship between societal discrimination and vulnerability to HIV. Mann (1993) states: 'The presence of discrimination against various groups within society has been identified as a major risk factor for HIV transmission'. He adds: 'It is obvious that if you belong to a discriminated-against group, you are less likely to benefit from AIDS programmes themselves, and from the information and services they provide'. He points out that people from such groups are less likely to have been involved in the design of AIDS informational campaigns, to recognize specific informational needs, and more likely to be subject to coercive and punitive measures.

It is clear that current national AIDS programmes provide a framework in which to plan and deliver a range of information, materials and services. In addition, discrimination has been identified as contributing to the difficulties in effectively targeting information and services at those who are discriminated against. What does not appear very clearly is what form discrimination takes. The debate over equity in health care will continue for the foreseeable future, with common, readily identifiable themes such as social status, cultural and religious beliefs, gender and sexuality issues. However, sweeping generalizations about 'groups' in society will not prove helpful in future planning. Grouping of clients has obvious disadvantages: for example, assumptions can be made that all members of a particular group participate in exactly the same behaviours or risk activities. We should perhaps work towards an elective approach, which assumes that individual members of 'groups' are likely to share at least some specific needs with the other members while maintaining their own individualistic needs. This approach can be helpful on a practitioner–client level but not in relation to resource allocation. In an analysis of national policies and strategies related to HIV/AIDS prevention, Cohen (1992) found that, while prevention was the main priority of national AIDS programmes, there was a remarkable lack of consistency between modes of transmission and the stages of the pandemic on the one hand, and the strategies, targeted groups and media choices on the other. Despite current evidence that interpersonal factors had the greatest impact on behaviour, many programmes devoted the majority of their funds to mass awareness programmes. In his study, Cohen also found that the least targeted, even in industrialized countries, were drug users, homosexual and bisexual men and immigrants.

THE UNITED KINGDOM RESPONSE

The Department of Health (DH) has been the leading agent for developing the British Government's overall planning strategy for HIV/AIDS. In 1986, the AIDS Unit was established within the DH to take on responsibility for developing a coherent and strategic approach to HIV and AIDS.

At a time when urgent action was needed, the Government responded by initiating a range of public health measures based on what was known about transmission. These included:

- protecting the UK blood supply;
- running a series of high-profile campaigns to inform the public about the risks of HIV infection and how they could be reduced;
- ensuring that young people received both formal and informal education about HIV;
- establishing harm reduction policies, such as needle exchange schemes, to counter the threat from HIV transmission associated with drug misuse.   (DH, 1993)

Earmarked monies for HIV/AIDS have been available since 1985 to encourage the development of NHS and local authority treatment and care services. NHS monies are distributed through regional health authorities to district health authorities who are required to account for expenditure for HIV/AIDS-related services. Since 1985, over £850 million has been made available to finance the UK AIDS programme which was underlined by a five-point strategy and coordinated across all departments.

The main thrust of the UK's AIDS strategy has been twofold:

1. to limit the further spread of HIV infection;
2. to provide diagnostic and treatment facilities as well as counselling and support services for those infected or at risk.

(DH, 1992)

To meet these objectives, the five-point strategy has comprised:

1. Prevention: to stem the spread of HIV infection through public awareness campaigns, community-based prevention initiatives, and improved infection control procedures;
2. Monitoring surveillance research: to improve understanding of the epidemiology of HIV infection, how it is transmitted, the natural history of the disease, and how HIV-related illness can be prevented and treated;
3. Treatment, care and support: to provide appropriate diagnostic, treatment, care and support services for those affected by HIV;
4. Social, legal and ethical issues: to foster a climate of understanding and compassion, to discourage discrimination and to safeguard confidentiality within the wider context of public health requirements;
5. International cooperation: to foster and encourage the full and continuing exchange of information between countries, and to encourage countries not to adopt coercive and discriminatory measures.

(DH, 1992)

Although the DH has never formally published a specific strategy document solely for HIV/AIDS, many documents and publications exist which, together, form the basis of a UK national AIDS programme/strategy. The DH has been assisted in this work by a number of groups set up to help central Government develop policies and priorities on HIV infection and AIDS (DH, 1992):

- The 'Expert Advisory Group on AIDS' (EAGA) is a group chaired by the Chief Medical Officer and comprises scientific and medical experts (including nursing representatives). Its remit is to provide advice to UK Chief Medical Officers on AIDS.
- The 'Interdepartmental Group on AIDS' (IDGA), whose membership is drawn from a wide range of Government departments with policy responsibilities affected by AIDS-related issues. The Group considers cross-departmental policy issues and exchanges information on developments.
- 'Coordination of AIDS Public Education' (CAPE), whose membership includes territorial health departments and their health education agencies, the Department of Education, the Foreign and Commonwealth Office, the Home Office, and the Health Education Authority. Its remit is to coordinate the public education efforts in the UK.

- The 'AIDS Services Working Group' (AWG), whose membership includes health services and local authority representatives. Its role is to advise the department on the implications of AIDS and HIV infection for the health and personal social services.
- The 'Chief Scientists' Group on AIDS Research', whose membership includes the Medical Research Council, Public Health Laboratory Services (PHLS), Economic and Social Research Council and the Department of Education. Its purpose is to identify gaps and overlaps in AIDS research programmes.

To spearhead the programme, the DH established an AIDS Unit in 1986, made up of a multiprofessional team with responsibility for monitoring and responding to the emerging HIV pandemic. In 1993, the AIDS Unit was integrated with other departments responsible for policy relating to communicable diseases. This new department is collectively known as the Communicable Diseases Branch.

PRIORITIZING FOR THE FUTURE

The Government's responses to HIV and AIDS have, in part, been informed by statistical data which aim to predict the incidence and prevalence of AIDS and HIV disease between specified dates.

A report from the Cox Committee (DH, 1988) had suggested that the incidence of AIDS in the UK would escalate to between 8000 and 34 077 cases by the end of 1992. This overestimated incidence added fuel to the fire that HIV/AIDS had become an 'industry', and as such was promulgated as a priority by AIDS activists and not by evidence from data (Stewart, 1993). In 1990, the Cox projections were revised down by Professor Nicholas Day, who suggested that there would be 3820 people alive with AIDS by the end of 1992 (PHLS, 1990). This figure proved to be a fairly accurate prediction.

In 1993, a working group led by Professor Day published new estimates for the period 1992–1997 (PHLS, 1993). This new study clearly demonstrates that reporting and monitoring systems are now far more sophisticated than they were. The collection of data from unlinked anonymous prevalence monitoring programmes, the greater length of time over which AIDS diagnoses have been reported, the higher volume of information on the effect of treatment on the incubation period, and the more powerful repertoire of analytical techniques, have all contributed to a significant reduction in the uncertainty of predicting the course of AIDS incidence over the past five years (PHLS, 1993). The estimates show a significantly lower figure for HIV infection and AIDS than previous reports have suggested.

In response to statistical evidence showing that HIV had reached a plateau in homosexual men, was declining among injecting drug users and steadily rising in the heterosexual population, the Government called for a review of policies to ensure that:

- resources were properly targeted;
- the right balance was struck with other health policies;
- HIV and AIDS were brought within the mainstream of health care and health promotion.

(DH, 1993)

STRATEGY FOR THE FUTURE

A Departmental Guidance Memorandum (1993), which was circulated throughout the statutory and non-statutory sectors indicated that 'four broad headings for HIV/AIDS work remain : prevention; treatment and care; monitoring, surveillance and research; and international action'.

The DH has reiterated its call for a concerted approach spanning Government, NHS, local authorities and the voluntary sector, including women's organizations, Britain's faith groups and organizations working with ethnic minorities, if the UK is to maintain 'this relatively favourable position' (DH, 1993). Prevention work will continue to be a priority area in terms of funding. It has been proposed that a greater focus on prevention should include efforts to:

- sustain and improve general public awareness, including for those who travel abroad;
- encourage appropriate behaviour change by increased targeting of sections of the population at particular risk, including homosexual and bisexual men and drug misusers;
- ensure that succeeding generations of children and young people continue to receive the information they need by working closely with the Department for Education, groups of parents, youth leaders and the media;
- safeguard the supply of blood, blood products and organs by screening through the transfusion service and by public education for potential donors;
- protect patients and staff by ensuring that published infection control and healthcare worker guidelines are well understood and implemented.

(DH, 1993)

Policies for the future in diagnosis, treatment and care will:

- continue to make HIV testing facilities more widely known and more readily available through primary care and other local resources;
- seek to influence the insurance industry so that their policies are consistent with public health requirements;
- ensure the provision of effective services for treatment and care in order to meet the changing needs of those affected by HIV and AIDS, including women, children, families and people from ethnic minorities, through reviewing health and local authority medical and social care;
- encourage the greater involvement of primary care staff by equipping them to give advice and information to patients;
- continue to support voluntary effort through funding.

(DH, 1993)

In relation to monitoring, surveillance and research, the DH will continue with its programme of anonymous HIV surveys and other studies for a more effective monitoring of the epidemic in order to facilitate resource allocation and service planning. International action will remain high profile through maintained and strengthened links with WHO and other international organizations aiming to limit the impact of the global epidemic.

As a result of the greater emphasis placed on mainstreaming HIV/AIDS, and following the calls for greater accountability over HIV/AIDS expenditure and for the right balance with other health priorities, the Government has been criticized and accused of listening to sceptics who do not believe that HIV is an urgent public health threat. Questions have been repeatedly asked about the high level of funding HIV/AIDS has attracted over the years. In 1993, with a cumulative total of 3000 cases (AIDS) alive today and an annual increase of 1500 cases, Stewart queried: 'Should AIDS be given priority in expenditure, institutional and community care over heart disease with over 200 000 deaths annually, or cancer with 100 000 deaths or an ageing population with all of these and much more?' Without doubt, it is becoming increasingly difficult to justify high levels of funding based on statistics alone. However, with the UK now having one of the lowest estimated HIV prevalence rates in western Europe, surely those critical of past high-level funding have to acknowledge that the UK's strategic approach has paid dividends in terms of low known levels of infection. Perhaps the anxieties voiced about withdrawal and the reduction of earmarked AIDS monies have more to do with the fear that HIV will be subsumed by other pressing health issues than with real concerns about the ability of generic services to effectively manage the care of individuals with HIV disease.

HEALTH OF THE NATION

In 1991, the Government published a discussion document 'The Health of the Nation', which set out proposals for the development of a health strategy for England. Included in the document was a series of key areas with clearly identified targets. It was proposed that the targets should provide an overall goal and sense of purpose; be explicit, quantified and monitorable over time through appropriate indicators; be achievable over a specified time; and be challenging (DH, 1992).

'The Health of the Nation' was seen as an important step in setting out attainable goals to improve the span of healthy life and was viewed as the UK's attempt to 'reorientate policies and programmes towards health rather than simply health care' (DH, 1992). The need for a shift in focus to promotion of health was something WHO had advocated in May 1977, when the World Health Assembly resolved that 'the main social target of governments and WHO in the coming decades should be the attainment by all citizens of the world by the year 2000 of a level of health that will permit them to lead a socially and economically productive life' (Resolution WHA30.43).

In July 1992 the Government published the White Paper 'Health of the Nation'. HIV/AIDS and sexual health had been included as a key area and was seen by those working in the field as an important step which further supported efforts to date. General objectives were laid out, together with specific targets. These were:

General objectives:
- to reduce the incidence of HIV infection;
- to reduce the incidence of other sexually transmitted diseases;
- to develop further and strengthen monitoring and surveillance;
- to provide effective services for diagnosis and treatment of HIV and other STDs;
- to reduce the number of unwanted pregnancies;
- to ensure the provision of effective family planning services for those people who want them.

Specific targets:

- to reduce the incidence of gonorrhoea among men and women aged 15–64 by at least 20% by 1995 (from 61 new cases per 100 000 population in 1990 to no more than 49 new cases per 100 000);
- to reduce the rate of conceptions among the under 16s by at least 50% by the year 2000 (from 9.5 per 1000 girls aged 13–15 in 1989 to no more than 4.8);
- to reduce the percentage of injecting drug misusers who report sharing injecting equipment in the previous four weeks by at least 50% by 1997, and by at least a further 50% by the year 2000 (from 20% in 1990 to no more than 10% by 1997, and no more than 5% by the year 2000).

(DH, 1993f)

The UK's strategic approach to HIV and AIDS has without doubt been complemented and strengthened by the launch of *'Health of the Nation'*. However, in the main, HIV and AIDS services are still viewed as the responsibility of 'specialist' workers. The UK Government's current efforts to 'mainstream' HIV and AIDS care will require all nurses to re-examine their current practice and identify, both individually and as a professional group, deficits in information, knowledge and skill.

THE NURSING RESPONSE

Research on nurses' knowledge and attitudes to HIV/AIDS is well documented (Bond *et al.*, 1989; Akinsanya and Rouse, 1991; McHaffie, 1993; Sharpe *et al.*, 1993). The research findings have caused great concern over the past few years and suggest that, as a professional group, nurses have not responded adequately to the challenge of HIV and AIDS. This is true in part, but some caution is called for inasmuch as these highly publicized research findings could undermine and overshadow admirable examples of HIV-related nursing practice. Throughout the country, many nurses have been proactive in establishing and evaluating a range of services for clients and patients affected by HIV. This has resulted in the development of models of care which have adequately met the needs of a range of client groups (Scott, 1994).

NURSING NETWORKS

The sharing and exchange of information has been a central and fundamental issue in developing HIV-related nursing practices. Many groups of nurses have realized the potential advantages of establishing forums for debate, discussion and exchange of information and ideas on HIV and AIDS. In 1990, a group of nurses from Denmark working in AIDS care organized a European conference for nurses which attracted over 220 delegates from 22 different countries. Subsequent conferences have been held in The Netherlands, Scotland, Hungary, Ireland and Spain. One consequence of these conferences has been the establishment of the European Association of Nurses in AIDS Care (EANAC). Although there have been problems in securing a financial base and effective administrative systems for EANAC, the annual conferences have provided opportunities for nurses from Europe to come together and share their experiences of responding to HIV and AIDS.

The Association of Nurses in Substance Abuse (ANSA) is a UK-based organization which has been instrumental in ensuring that drug use and HIV issues remain high on the nursing agenda. Annual conferences, regional meetings and a regular journal have contributed to the effective dissemination of information and examples of good practice. Similarly, the Royal College of Nursing's HIV Nursing Forum has served as a network which aims to support and inform practitioners in their work. More recently, the Genito-Urinary Nurses Association (GUNA) has been established and aims to strengthen mechanisms for support and information exchange on a range of issues, such as nursing patients with sexually transmitted diseases (STDs), or HIV and sexual health.

Nurse educationalists responsible for English National Board (ENB) HIV and AIDS courses have been supported in their work through the Board's HIV and AIDS Education and Training Project (ENB, 1994). Annual workshops for nurse educationalists took place between 1990 and 1993, and have since been organized and facilitated by a London-based college of nursing.

These are just some examples of what steps have been taken over the past few years to disseminate information and increase access to support and research findings in the field of HIV, AIDS and drug misuse. However, a critical analysis of the situation would suggest that these forums are geared to the needs of the specialist worker and not readily accessible to the wider profession. The need for such organizations is self-evident, but there is a danger that they will continue to reinforce the perception that HIV, AIDS, drug use and sexual health remain the responsibility of the `specialist' worker. Perhaps these organizations need to take stock of their aims and objectives, review their mechanisms for disseminating information and find ways of making themselves more 'attractive' to the wider profession. In addition, more time needs to be devoted to developing systems for supporting the 'non-specialist' worker in HIV-related work.

CHALLENGES FOR THE FUTURE

The challenges for the future in HIV-related nursing practice are many. Nurses will need to closely examine the needs of individuals and groups, both those infected and directly affected by HIV and those who are not (although this is a debatable point). WHO (1992) propose that the new challenges of the evolving pandemic are:

- increased emphasis on care;
- better treatment for other sexually transmitted diseases;
- greater focus on HIV prevention through improvement of women's health, educational, legal and social status;
- a more supportive environment for prevention programmes;
- provision for the socioeconomic impact of the pandemic;
- greater emphasis on explaining the public health dangers of stigmatization and discrimination.

Beedham and Wilson-Barnett (1993) suggested that the needs of people with HIV and AIDS did not differ significantly from the needs of other diagnostic groups. However, a number of factors were thought to influence the needs of such people and to differentiate between HIV/AIDS and other chronic illnesses. They reported that the stigma associated with HIV and AIDS resulted in prejudice, ostracism, harassment and oppression. Mann (1993) proposes that one of the main challenges for health and social care professionals is to undertake a systematic review of existing HIV/AIDS programmes to identify those forms of discrimination that exist in them. He asks: 'Are our informational programmes reaching those whom we need to reach? Is the necessary mix of services and support available truly accessible to those who need them? And are there marginalized groups in society who remain outside the community and national AIDS efforts?'

The provision of a quality nursing service for people affected by or infected with HIV will require all nurses to critically evaluate current practice. There are policy frameworks and guidance for ensuring quality in nursing practice at international, national, regional and local levels. Structures are in place for nurses to tailor their practice to meet the needs of individuals, groups, communities and society at large. Key documents, such as: *A Strategy for Nursing* (DH, 1989b); *A Vision for the Future* (DH, 1993d); *Caring for People* (DH, 1989a); *Targeting Practice – The Contribution of Nurses, Midwives and Health Visitors to The Health of the*

Nation (DH, 1993c); *Ethnicity and Health* (DH, 1993a); *The Scope of Professional Practice* (UKCC, 1992); *New World, New Opportunities – Nursing in Primary Health Care* (DH, 1993b) and *The Global AIDS Strategy* (WHO, 1992) provide an extensive and in-depth view on how nursing will develop health-care provision and respond to HIV and AIDS over the next decade. However, it is somewhat presumptuous and naïve to think that the challenges of HIV will be addressed by policy frameworks and guidance alone. Taerk *et al.* (1993) state that there are tremendous pressures exerted on health-care workers to care empathically for people with AIDS, pointing to the consensus of opinion that health-care workers have 'bad' attitudes in relation to HIV and AIDS. Education and training remain the key to empower and equip nurses with sufficient knowledge, information and opportunities for developing skills to rise to the challenge of HIV and AIDS effectively: 'It appears that changing attitudes of health-care workers from bad ones to good ones addresses only a part of the problem. In fact, alone this philosophy can be counterproductive. What is clearly needed, in addition to attempting to change attitudes of health professionals, is an understanding and acknowledgement of the legitimacy of staff concerns (i.e. contagion, homophobia and attachment and loss)' (Taerk *et al.*, 1993). It seems that the challenge of HIV to the nursing profession amounts to much more than developing user-friendly, accessible and appropriate services. Human rights and social justice have been highlighted as the key issues of a strategy for the future. Mann (1993) proposes that health workers should 'reach out beyond their traditional colleagues – to collaborate directly with groups engaged in increasing social justice and promoting human rights'. This approach would require nurses to enter into new styles of dialogue with agencies and politically activated bodies. As Jolley (1989) comments: 'There is a continuing need for nurses to become more politically aware. In failing to do so, they fail their patients and themselves, while others outside nursing, as so often in the past, make the decisions for them.' Given that many nurses are politically naïve and unmotivated, and that for many HIV and AIDS is not a priority, promoting human rights and increasing social justice is not a role that will be readily taken on board. Perhaps one solution would be to enable nurses, through more explicit education and training on the issue, to identify how discrimination affects access to health care generally. If time allows, only then will the lessons learnt be transferable to the growing public health issue of HIV and AIDS.

'The optimist proclaims that we live in the best of all possible worlds; and the pessimist fears this is true.' (Source unknown)

REFERENCES

Akinsanya, J.A. and Rouse, P. (1991) *Who Will Care? A Survey of the Knowledge and Attitudes of Hospital Nurses to People with HIV/AIDS.* Anglia Polytechnic Faculty of Health and Social Work, Chelmsford.

Beedham, H.M. and Wilson-Barnett, J. (1993) Evaluation of services for people with HIV/AIDS in an inner city health authority: perspectives of key service providers. *Journal of Advanced Nursing*, **18**, 69–79.

Bond, S. *et al.* (1989) *A National Study of HIV Infection, AIDS and Community Nursing Staff in England. A Summary of A Report.* Health Care Research Unit, University of Newcastle upon Tyne.

Cohen, M., Tarantola, D., Netter, T. *et al.* (1992) Worldwide Responses to HIV Prevention. Paper presented to the VIIIth International Conference on AIDS/STDS World Congress, Amsterdam, The Netherlands, 19–24 July 1992.

Crawley, R.H. (1988) Introduction, in *AIDS: Psychiatric and Psychosocial Perspectives* (ed. L. Paine). Croom Helm, London.

Decosas, J. (1993) Cited in Kirby, M. Colloquium on AIDS, Health and Human Rights, Foundation Marcel Merieux, Institut des Sciences du Vivant, Annecy, France, 18–20 June 1993. *AIDS Care*, 6(2), 247–52, 1994.

Department of Health (1988) *Short Term Prediction of HIV Infection and AIDS in England and Wales. Report of a Working Group* (The Cox Report). HMSO, London.

Department of Health (1989a) *Caring for People: Community Care in the Next Decade and Beyond.* HMSO, London.

Department of Health (1989b) *A Strategy for Nursing: Report of the Steering Committee.* HMSO, London.

Department of Health (1992a) *Health of the Nation: A Strategy for Health for England.* HMSO, London.

Department of Health (1992b) *AIDS Briefing Note* (Unpublished). DH, London.

Department of Health (1993a) *Ethnicity and Health: A Guide for the NHS.* HMSO, London.

Department of Health (1993b) *New World, New Opportunities: Nursing in Primary Health Care.* HMSO, London.

Department of Health (1993c) *Targeting Practice: The Contribution of Nurses, Midwives and Health Visitors. Health of the Nation.* HMSO, London.

Department of Health (1993d) *A Vision for the Future: The Nursing, Midwifery and Health Visiting Contribution to Health and Health Care.* HMSO, London.

Department of Health (1993e) *Government Strategy on HIV and AIDS* (unpublished). DH, London.

Department of Health (1993f) *Key Area Handbook on HIV and Sexual Health: Health of the Nation.* HMSO, London.

English National Board (1994) *The HIV/AIDS Education and Training Project 1990–1994: A Report.* ENB, London.

Global AIDS Policy Coalition (1993) *Towards a New Health Strategy for AIDS. A Report.* The Global AIDS Policy Coalition, USA.

Jolley, M. (1989) *Current Issues in Nursing.* Chapman & Hall, London.

Mann, J.M. (1993) AIDS policy in evolution: learning from experience, in *Report of the 1993 Conference of European Community Paliamentarians on HIV/AIDS,*

23–24 April 1993, London. British All-Party Parliamentary Groups on AIDS, United Kingdom.

McHaffie, H. (1993) *The care of patients with HIV and AIDS: a survey of nurse education in the UK: A Report.* Institute of Medical Ethics, University of Edinburgh, Edinburgh.

Merson, M.H. (1992) Foreword to: *WHO, The Global AIDS Strategy.* WHO, Geneva.

Merson, M.H. (1994) The HIV/AIDS Pandemic: Global Status of the HIV/AIDS Epidemic and the Response. Plenary Presentation to the Xth International Conference on AIDS, 7–11 August 1994, Yokohama, Japan.

PHLS (1990) *Acquired Immune Deficiency Syndrome in England and Wales to end 1993: projections using data to end September 1989.* Report of a working group convened by the Director of the Public Health Laboratory Service (The Day Report). Communicable Disease Report 1990 (suppl).

PHLS (1993) *The Incidence and Prevalence of AIDS and Other Severe HIV Disease in England and Wales for 1992–1997: Projections using data to the end of June 1992.* Report of a Working Group. Communicable Disease Report 1993; 3 (suppl 1): S1–17.

Scott, C. (1994) *The Care and Treatment of People with HIV Disease and AIDS: A Nursing Perspective.* Royal College of Nursing, London.

Sharpe, C., Maychell, K. and Walton, I. (1993) *Nursing and AIDS: Material Matters.* Issues, Information and Teaching Materials on HIV and AIDS for Nurses (A Research Study). National Foundation for Educational Research, Slough.

Stewart, G. (1993) Predictable and preventable? *Nursing Times,* **89**(26), 29–32.

Taerk, R.M. *et al.* (1993) Recurrent Themes of Concern in Groups of Health Professionals. *AIDS Care,* **5**(2), 215–21.

UKCC (1992) *The Scope of Professional Practice.* UKCC, London.

World Health Organization (1978) *Alma Ata 1978: Report of the International Conference on Primary Health Care: Health for All by the Year 2000,* Resolution WHA30.43. WHO, Geneva.

World Health Organization (1985) *Targets for Health for All.* WHO, Geneva.

World Health Organization (1986) *The Global AIDS Strategy.* WHO, Geneva.

World Health Organization (1992) *The Global AIDS Strategy.* WHO, Geneva.

HIV/AIDS research evidence – dilemmas and lessons in a multiprofessional context

2

Jean Faugier and Ian Hicken

INTRODUCTION

During the past decade AIDS and HIV have come to constitute a unique challenge to a number of professional groups, as those currently working in this field have had to learn quickly how to adapt to each new situation and how best to manage the provision of care for their particular group of clients in order to ensure a high-quality service. While much excellent knowledge has been gained in this way, leading to the provision of exemplary care, the current situation is far from ideal: indeed, there is equal weight of evidence to show that many staff, lacking confidence and knowledge, are ill prepared to deal with their clients' needs.

If we are to ensure with a greater degree of certainty that clients receive the best possible response to the complexity of physical, social and psychological problems associated with AIDS and HIV, we need to examine the research evidence available to us and attempt to make suitable changes to the provision of future professional training, practice and supervision.

In this chapter the research findings that relate to nursing practice and education will be considered. The chapter will also examine how current provision of care and training in HIV/AIDS has attempted to meet the needs outlined in the research as well as indicate those particular issues that require future strategic planning initiatives.

THE RESEARCH EVIDENCE

In the last 5 years a number of important research reports examining various professional groups and their role in relation to AIDS have been funded and have become widely available. The majority of these studies focused on experiences and attitudes in relation to AIDS, and did not specifically set out to investigate the needs of nurses as a particular professional group; nevertheless, they provide some very important messages for future strategies. In addition, other studies examining the behaviour of specific client groups have also highlighted the need for more, or improved, professional training and an improved response from nurses generally.

THE MAJOR THEMES

In reporting their findings the various researchers identified a number of central themes as major areas of concern for professional training. These constitute important components of quality practice and training in the field of HIV and AIDS. However, the findings from the research reports are not limited to messages aimed at those seeking to provide specialist courses in HIV and AIDS; they also contain very clear pointers to the deficiencies of current professional training in a range of vital areas.

ATTITUDES

In the first major study of HIV/AIDS and community nursing undertaken by Bond et al. (1988), negative attitudes to those who became infected were found to be a possible factor in the unwillingness or inability of community nurses to cope with the challenge of HIV. More than a quarter of nurses surveyed considered that they should have the right to refuse to care for a patient with AIDS, and more than a fifth felt that they should have the right to refuse to care for those who are HIV positive. Of particular concern was the finding that one in every four midwives considered, either positively or with a degree of uncertainty about it, that they should have the right to refuse care for those with HIV/AIDS. The evidence from studies of nurses working in inpatient settings is equally disturbing: in a study of hospital nursing staff, Akinsanya et al. (1991) found that 37% of a randomly selected sample of 717 hospital nurses from 11 health authorities believed they should also have the right to refuse to deliver care to those infected with HIV. These findings indicated a substantial body of opinion in community nursing at odds with the code of professional conduct issued by the United Kingdom Central Council for Nursing, Midwifery and Health Visiting (UKCC, 1990). Findings from these research projects have stimulated further official pronouncements from the UKCC concerning the 'duty to care'.

A study of general practitioners by Gallagher *et al.* (1989) reported similar findings, with 6% of the sample saying they did not wish to deliver care to patients on their list who might develop AIDS, and a further 20% expressing doubts about doing so.

Apart from a fear of HIV itself and condemnation of individuals' lifestyles, other factors have been shown to influence the willingness to engage with patients infected with HIV. In an evaluation of a series of workshops for senior community nursing managers, Robottom (1989) reported that staff working in low-prevalence areas were failing to give appropriate time and resources to HIV, arguing instead that they had other areas of concern deserving of priority. Robinson *et al.* (1991a), in a study of social work preparation for HIV/AIDS conducted as part of the Landmark evaluation, also reported particular problems related to low-prevalence areas, and found managers commonly reporting difficulties in motivating staff who had not yet had any referrals.

Social service managers also reported difficulties in raising interest and awareness of HIV/AIDS issues in staff who perceived themselves to be underresourced for their current client demand.

The presence of such attitudes, combined with the very real demands of HIV, has led to the development of a range of specialist services, in particular specialist nursing teams and home support teams. McCann and Wadsworth (1991) found that access to such a team was regarded extremely positively by clients, who perceived their needs as being more effectively met by such specialists. In particular, such teams are viewed as islands of protection for vulnerable client groups from the assault of negative attitudes which the earlier research uncovered. Such specialism, however, can ultimately act as a barrier to the accessibility of appropriate generic support services for those with HIV/AIDS. Robinson *et al.* (1991a) found that 85% of a sample of those with HIV/AIDS agreed with the statement that 'It is better for services to be provided by those who specialize in HIV work rather than those with general workloads'. They felt that specialists would be better trained to understand the needs and feelings of people with the virus.

Preliminary findings from research into the provision of generic community nursing services for those with HIV/AIDS found that specialist teams were often reluctant to refer clients to generic staff, whose attitudes they perceived to be negative. This was particularly true in the early stages of the epidemic, when such attitudes were being expressed and acted on by generic staff.

These early findings, reported by Butterworth *et al.* (1993), do, however, provide evidence that attitudes change significantly with experience. District nurse respondents to the study identified their major concerns prior to their first HIV/AIDS patient as focusing on three main areas of concern:

- Lack of knowledge and experience to care: This related mainly to concerns about well-informed patients, lack of access to up-to-date information about the disease, and lack of support.
- Certain aspects of HIV-related care: This primarily related to the emotional aspects of caring for someone with HIV disease, concern that the protective clothing they thought they would need might be stigmatizing and offensive to patients, and concern that care at home might be too complex to manage.
- Concerns regarding the disease itself: Fear of contracting the virus during a procedure, being unfamiliar with the symptoms of the disease, nursing homosexual patients, and nursing someone with a sexually transmitted disease.

When the nurses were asked to identify their major concerns following experience of nursing someone with HIV, they fell into the following main areas:

- problems of updating one's knowledge, especially with regard to new treatments;
- lack of training in skills such as counselling and bereavement counselling;
- lack of time to devote to nursing patients and to providing support to significant others.

As is obvious, although there are still indications of concern about skills, these are now expressed in a positive vein and relate to specific deficiencies rather than to HIV in particular. Unfortunately, however, the reputation earned by generic primary health-care staff for poor attitudes in the early stages of the epidemic has provided a barrier to effective utilization of such staff in many regions.

Negative attitudes have been shown to be particularly strong and more resistant to change when they relate to drug users, who are perceived to be particularly difficult or undesirable. Many studies – Gallagher *et al.* (1989); Robinson *et al.* (1991b); Wadsworth and McCann (1992); Faugier *et al.* (1992) – have indicated that negative attitudes towards this client group are militating against access to a range of important health-care and preventive services.

Training for all professional groups must first and foremost address any attitude problems that exist, allow professionals to express such feelings in a safe environment, and proceed to identify ways forward. Such training methods should not be reserved specifically for HIV/AIDS courses but should be incorporated into basic and post-basic professional training, and expanded to cover a wider range of issues to which they are equally relevant. Such an approach, tested and evaluated by Sibbald *et al.* (1991), showed positive attitude changes in groups of GPs and practice nurses when they had been provided with an opportunity to improve their knowledge, attitudes and skills.

CONTACT WITH PATIENTS

The amount of contact professionals have with those infected with HIV is important in determining confidence and fostering positive attitudes. A number of studies have provided evidence which suggests that theoretical input alone appears to be insufficient in bringing about the professional confidence required to ensure high-quality care. Having role models available within an organization, or training experience against which trainees may measure their responses, is of obvious importance.

The work of Bond *et al.* (1989) suggests, however, that limited experience of HIV does not by itself result in greater nursing staff confidence to deliver input in relation to health education, counselling on sexual issues and terminal care. At the time of the Bond survey, only 4.1% of the sample had dealt with a client with AIDS, and this contact was frequently limited to individual patients on any caseload. This situation has changed considerably and many more community nurses now have experience of nursing those with HIV/AIDS. In a study of generic district nursing staff providing care for those with HIV, Brocklehurst *et al.* (1993) found a significant change in perceptions. Similarly, Gallagher *et al.* (1989) also found limited contact with people with AIDS among the GPs in their study. Only 6.4% of practitioners knew of patients in the practice who had AIDS, although more knew of others who were asymptomatic. As might be expected, there were wide geographical variations and, while the majority of GPs expressed a willingness to provide care for those on their list who might become infected with HIV, the majority were unwilling to do so for injecting drug users (or even to register them).

Evidence from other studies of GPs' attitudes to injecting drug users suggests that such an unwillingness has little to do with associated HIV infection, but is more likely to be the result of lack of confidence among GPs and a perception of inadequate professional support when working with this client group.

There are enormous implications in these findings for the work and importance of practice nurses in acting as a bridge for the client to appropriate and sensitive care.

KNOWLEDGE OF HIV INFECTION

Several studies have exposed the inadequacy of knowledge in relation to HIV/AIDS among various professional groups. In one of the early studies, Bond *et al.* (1989) reported a disappointing lack of knowledge among all disciplines of community nursing staff. In particular, staff made incorrect and potentially dangerous judgements as to the extent of risk of infection. Respondents were much more likely to overestimate the possibility of infection from needlestick injuries and contact with contaminated blood or body fluids. Although such an overestimation has a protective function for nursing staff, it carries possibilities of stigmatization for those infected with the virus.

Forty per cent of nursing staff reported a concern over their lack of knowledge, which was further supported by the results of a multiple-choice test. There was, however, a small but significant difference between those staff reporting that they had dealt with HIV infection and/or who had attended in-service training on HIV infection, and those who had had no experience of either of these two inputs.

Throughout the findings, the insecurity of community nurses about their knowledge and experience of HIV infections are only too evident. Of greatest concern was the fact that there seemed to be very little transfer of existing knowledge and skills. Many of the nursing procedures and responsibilities in respect of those with HIV/AIDS are identical, or similar, to the work undertaken by community nurses with other patients on their caseload.

The research findings from the studies of hospital nurses by Bond *et al.* (1989), and more recently Akinsanya and Rouse (1991), provided scant evidence of the utilization of existing skills and knowledge when approaching the problems posed by HIV/AIDS. Especially concerning were the findings reported by Bond and Rhodes (1990) that community midwives demonstrated a limited knowledge of HIV infection and that almost two-thirds of the respondents to their study were worried about keeping up to date with trends and developments. The Akinsanya study raises particularly alarming findings about the level of knowledge hospital nurses have about the possibility of infection and their consequent rights to have access to the test results and details of patients' HIV status: 57% of nurses surveyed felt that the result of an HIV test should be made available to all staff. There was a completely false estimation of risk of infection, arising not only from professional contact with those infected by HIV but also from everyday domestic contact.

In their study of HIV/AIDS and general practice, Gallagher *et al.* (1989) showed that most practitioners were aware that the procedures for avoiding hepatitis B infection are also appropriate for avoiding HIV infection. However, there was a degree of confusion about the risk of acquiring HIV from a needlestick injury, an uncertainty with regard to the wearing of gloves and the need to abandon the practice of resheathing needles. Over a quarter of GPs wrongly assessed the risk of acquiring HIV after a needlestick injury, and a fifth of them were uncertain about this risk. It was alarming to note that, although three out of five doctors had a policy of wearing gloves when taking blood, over a quarter had decided against resheathing needles or were uncertain about doing so. Practitioners were lacking in knowledge of symptoms and signs of HIV-related illness and AIDS and, significantly, the majority of GPs had not seen it as relevant to produce a practice policy in relation to HIV/AIDS clinical management, infection control and referral to other services.

In a study of GP trainers and trainees by Brown-Peterside *et al.* (1991), the proportion of doctors scoring more than 5 out of 10 in a knowledge assessment was significantly higher among trainees than trainers. In a study of 263 HIV-positive homosexual men, Wadsworth and McCann (1992) found that a major reason for underuse of GP facilities by this group was a lack of confidence in the GPs' knowledge and understanding of HIV; additionally, patients were fearful of breach of confidentiality and stigmatizing treatment by GPs unfamiliar with the needs of those infected with HIV. Nurses working as members of the primary health-care team will need to confront these issues with medical colleagues in a manner which facilitates change and which emphasizes the role of the nurse as the 'advocate' for equitable and ethical treatment.

SEXUALITY AND SEXUAL BEHAVIOUR

A wide range of research studies undertaken so far have demonstrated a lack of skill and confidence among professional workers when raises particularly alarming findings about the level of knowledge hospital nurses have about the possibility of infection and the consequent rights to have access to the test results and details of patients' HIV status: 57% of nurses surveyed felt that the result of a HIV test should be made available to all staff. There was a completely false estimation of risk of infection, arising not only from professional contact with those infected by HIV but also from everyday domestic contact.

In their study of HIV/AIDS and general practice, Gallagher et al. (1989) showed that most practitioners were aware that the procedures for avoiding hepatitis B infection are also appropriate for avoiding HIV infection. However, there was a degree of confusion about the risk of acquiring HIV from a needlestick injury, an uncertainty with regard to the wearing of gloves and the need to abandon the practice of resheathing needles. Over a quarter of GPs wrongly assessed the risk of acquiring HIV after a needlestick injury, and a fifth of them were uncertain about this risk. It was alarming to note that, although three out of five doctors had a policy of wearing gloves when taking blood, over a quarter had decided against resheathing needles or were uncertain about doing so. Practitioners were lacking in knowledge of symptoms and signs of HIV-related illness and AIDS and, significantly, the majority of GPs had not seen it as relevant to produce a practice policy in relation to HIV/AIDS clinical management, infection control and referral to other services.

In a study of GP trainers and trainees by Brown-Peterside et al. (1991), the proportion of doctors scoring more than 5 out of 10 in a knowledge assessment was significantly higher among trainees than trainers. In a study of 263 HIV-positive homosexual men, Wadsworth and McCann (1992) found that a major reason for underuse of GP facilities by this group was a lack of confidence in the GPs' knowledge and understanding of HIV; additionally, patients were fearful of breach of confidentiality and stigmatizing treatment by GPs unfamiliar with the needs of those infected with HIV. Nurses working as members of the primary health-care team will need to confront these issues with medical colleagues in a manner which facilitates change and which emphasizes the role of the nurse as the 'advocate' for equitable and ethical treatment.

SEXUALITY AND SEXUAL BEHAVIOUR

A wide range of research studies undertaken so far have demonstrated a lack of skill and confidence among professional workers when in the early stages of the epidemic, when such attitudes were being expressed and acted on by generic staff.

These early findings, reported by Butterworth et al. (1993), do, however, provide evidence that attitudes change significantly with experience. District nurse respondents to the study identified their major concerns prior to their first HIV/AIDS patient as focusing on three main areas of concern:

- Lack of knowledge and experience to care: This related mainly to concerns about well-informed patients, lack of access to up-to-date information about the disease, and lack of support.
- Certain aspects of HIV-related care: This primarily related to the emotional aspects of caring for someone with HIV disease, concern that the protective clothing they thought they would need might be stigmatizing and offensive to patients, and concern that care at home might be too complex to manage.
- Concerns regarding the disease itself: Fear of contracting the virus during a procedure, being unfamiliar with the symptoms of the disease, nursing homosexual patients, and nursing someone with a sexually transmitted disease.

When the nurses were asked to identify their major concerns following experience of nursing someone with HIV, they fell into the following main areas:

- problems of updating one's knowledge, especially with regard to new treatments;
- lack of training in skills such as counselling and bereavement counselling;
- lack of time to devote to nursing patients and to providing support to significant others.

As is obvious, although there are still indications of concern about skills, these are now expressed in a positive vein and relate to specific deficiencies rather than to HIV in particular. Unfortunately, however, the reputation earned by generic primary health-care staff for poor attitudes in the early stages of the epidemic has provided a barrier to effective utilization of such staff in many regions.

Negative attitudes have been shown to be particularly strong and more resistant to change when they relate to drug users, who are perceived to be particularly difficult or undesirable. Many studies – Gallagher et al. (1989); Robinson et al. (1991b); Wadsworth and McCann (1992); Faugier et al. (1992) – have indicated that negative attitudes towards this client group are militating against access to a range of important health-care and preventive services.

Training for all professional groups must first and foremost address any attitude problems that exist, allow professionals to express such feelings in a safe environment, and proceed to identify ways forward. Such training methods should not be reserved specifically for HIV/AIDS courses but should be incorporated into basic and post-basic professional training, and expanded to cover a wider range of issues to which they are equally relevant. Such an approach, tested and evaluated by Sibbald et al. (1991), showed positive attitude changes in groups of GPs and practice nurses when they had been provided with an opportunity to improve their knowledge, attitudes and skills.

CONTACT WITH PATIENTS

The amount of contact professionals have with those infected with HIV is important in determining confidence and fostering positive attitudes. A number of studies have provided evidence which suggests that theoretical input alone appears to be insufficient in bringing about the professional confidence required to ensure high-quality care. Having role models available within an organization, or training experience against which trainees may measure their responses, is of obvious importance.

The work of Bond et al. (1989) suggests, however, that limited experience of HIV does not by itself result in greater nursing staff confidence to deliver input in relation to health education, counselling on sexual issues and terminal care. At the time of the Bond survey, only 4.1% of the sample had dealt with a client with AIDS, and this contact was frequently limited to individual patients on any caseload. This situation has changed considerably and many more community nurses now have experience of nursing those with HIV/AIDS. In a study of generic district nursing staff providing care for those with HIV, Brocklehurst et al. (1993) found a significant change in perceptions. Similarly, Gallagher et al. (1989) also found limited contact with people with AIDS among the GPs in their study. Only 6.4% of practitioners knew of patients in the practice who had AIDS, although more knew of others who were asymptomatic. As might be expected, there were wide geographical variations and, while the majority of GPs expressed a willingness to provide care for those on their list who might become infected with HIV, the majority were unwilling to do so for injecting drug users (or even to register them).

Evidence from other studies of GPs' attitudes to injecting drug users suggests that such an unwillingness has little to do with associated HIV infection, but is more likely to be the result of lack of confidence among GPs and a perception of inadequate professional support when working with this client group.

There are enormous implications in these findings for the work and importance of practice nurses in acting as a bridge for the client to appropriate and sensitive care.

KNOWLEDGE OF HIV INFECTION

Several studies have exposed the inadequacy of knowledge in relation to HIV/AIDS among various professional groups. In one of the early studies, Bond et al. (1989) reported a disappointing lack of knowledge among all disciplines of community nursing staff. In particular, staff made incorrect and potentially dangerous judgements as to the extent of risk of infection. Respondents were much more likely to overestimate the possibility of infection from needlestick injuries and contact with contaminated blood or body fluids. Although such an overestimate has a protective function for nursing staff, it carries possibilities of stigmatization for those infected with the virus.

Forty per cent of nursing staff reported a concern over their lack of knowledge, which was further supported by the results of a multiple choice test. There was, however, a small but significant difference between those staff reporting that they had dealt with HIV infection and/or who had attended in-service training on HIV infection, and those who had had no experience of either of these two inputs.

Throughout the findings, the insecurity of community nurses about their knowledge and experience of HIV infections are only too evident. Of greatest concern was the fact that there seemed to be very little transfer of existing knowledge and skills. Many of the new procedures and responsibilities in respect of those with HIV/AIDS identical, or similar, to the work undertaken by community nurses with other patients on their caseload.

The research findings from the studies of hospital nurses by Bond et al. (1989), and more recently Akinsanya and Rouse (1991), provide scant evidence of the utilization of existing skills and knowledge in approaching the problems posed by HIV/AIDS. Especially concerning were the findings reported by Bond and Rhodes (1990) that community midwives demonstrated a limited knowledge of HIV infection and almost two-thirds of the respondents to their study were worried about keeping up to date with trends and developments. The Akinsanya confronted with issues related to sexuality. Stimson *et al.* (1989) found staff employed in syringe exchange settings reluctant or unable to counsel drug users about their sexual behaviour. A study by Faugier *et al.* (1992) of female drug-using prostitutes displayed similar concerns about the lack of readiness and preparedness on the part of community drug teams and primary health-care staff to counsel their clients on sexual issues. A majority of the female respondents to the study had been in contact with maternity services at some stage; however, there was little, if any, evidence that an opportunity had been taken by nursing and midwifery staff to provide sexual health education or counselling.

Bond *et al.* (1989) reported that the discussion of sexual matters relating to HIV infection created much more unease among community nursing staff than did sexual health education related to other topics. Surprisingly, in a national study of genitourinary medicine clinics, Allen and Hogg (1993) also point to the need for increased confidence among nurses and health advisers working in such settings in relation to sexual counselling and health education. The impression from the research is that HIV and the fears it generates seem somehow to get in the way of the effective use of existing skills. HIV counselling and related sexual counselling appears to have more mystery attached to it than does other work, and the emphasis placed on the need to limit the spread of infection has to some extent made the discussion of the nature of transmission, or the nature of drug misuse, more dominant than any discussion of basic sexual risk behaviour.

It is perhaps the universality of such sexual behaviour which is threatening and uncomfortable to those professionals charged with the task of providing counselling and advice. The additional challenge of accepting and coming to terms with the sexuality of others is something that most professionals express a need to be prepared for.

Homosexual respondents to the Wadsworth and McCann study clearly identify this fear of rejection of their sexual lifestyle by the GP as a reason for underuse of primary health-care services. Additionally, in a study of informal carers by McCann and Wadsworth (1992), the ability of such carers to accept the sexuality and lifestyle of a person with AIDS was shown to be important in the provision of physical and emotional care. This discomfort was confirmed by Brown *et al.*, who found that trainee GPs expressed difficulty in discussing sexual issues and behaviour with all types of patients, but had the greatest difficulty with homosexuals. The researchers also point to a lack of confidence in delivering counselling to HIV-positive patients and a reluctance to elicit sexual histories; this is of immense concern when one considers that the skills involved are fundamental to the work in general practice and crucial to the provision of appropriate advice.

SUPPORT AND SUPERVISION

Much of the research displayed a lack of adequate support and supervision of professional staff in view of the new demands many of them felt were being made on their skills by the arrival of HIV/AIDS. Community nurses responding to the Bond and Rhodes (1990) survey expressed a lack of confidence in their managers' ability to provide appropriate support networks. The large majority of community nursing staff had also not had access to policy statements or guidance on a wide range of topics associated with HIV infection.

Similarly, the research by Gallagher *et al.* (1989) relating to GPs presents a picture of isolated practitioners functioning frequently in the absence of specific policy and practice guidelines.

INFECTION CONTROL AND CLINICAL PRACTICE

The research displays a real need for regular updates of infection control guidelines as they apply to the practice of professional workers. HIV infection is an illness with a rapidly changing knowledge base; this applies to its epidemiology, transmissibility and clinical management. All research studies indicate a relationship between clear specific knowledge and guidelines and the level of professional confidence in caring for those with HIV/AIDS.

Optimistically, the concern raised by HIV has heightened the awareness of clinical staff of the need to reassess the effectiveness of current infection control practices, particularly with regard to the standards appropriate to avoid the transmission of hepatitis B. However, as much of the research so far mentioned clearly demonstrates, there is considerable confusion, and no small measure of complacency, in these matters.

PREPARATION FOR, AND CONFIDENCE IN, COUNSELLING

Counselling is seen not only as a fundamental skill required by many health-care workers, but also as a major source of support and health education for those affected by, and at risk of, HIV. It is therefore of concern that a number of research reports – Bond *et al.* (1989); Allen and Hogg *et al.* (1993); Faugier *et al.* (1992); Gallagher *et al.* (1989); Robinson *et al.* (1991a) – identify lack of confidence and skill in this area. Once again, it would appear that HIV has either exposed a lack of confidence and skill, or has resulted in an inability to transfer fundamental professional skills to the care of those with HIV.

Of particular concern is the evidence which suggests that even those staff working on what might be considered the 'front line' in terms of HIV prevention, involved in pre- and post-test counselling, and counselling on sexual health education, should also display a lack of preparation and confidence to fulfil this role.

PROVIDING CARE FOR DRUG USERS

Evidence from a range of studies suggests that attitudes towards drug users, particularly those who inject, provide a serious barrier to providing appropriate accessible health care for this client group. Equally important is the perception expressed by injecting drug users that they are more than likely to face negative attitudes on the part of health-care workers displaying a judgemental approach to their behaviour or lifestyle. Gallagher *et al.* (1989) found that less than half the respondents to the survey wished to accept injecting drug users on to their practice list, on top of the 6% who would actively seek to remove such patients from their lists. In a study of drug-using prostitutes, Faugier *et al.* (1992) reported that a majority of the women had at some time been refused treatment by a GP.

Other professional groups, mainly nurses and pharmacists, have shown more willingness to engage in work with injecting drug users but do express a need for information and support. Glanz *et al.* (1990) found that community pharmacists saw themselves as having an important role to play while expressing reservations and concerns for the controls and boundaries to such involvement.

CIVIL RIGHTS AND CONFIDENTIALITY

Recent events which have involved infected health-care workers and media intrusion, frequently involving allegations of chequebook journalism, have given sharp focus to the ongoing debate about the right to confidentiality and the need to respect the civil rights of those with HIV. However, the research evidence would suggest that professional health-care workers had given little thought to these issues earlier in the epidemic.

A number of studies, most notably by Bond *et al.* (1989) and Akinsanya (1991), indicate a very worrying disregard for the civil rights of those with HIV/AIDS. Perhaps of even greater concern is the finding by Gallagher *et al.* (1989) that the majority of GPs who responded to their survey were in favour of divulging the HIV status to a wide range of other professionals without seeking the patient's consent; moreover,

37% were in favour of testing without consent for injecting drug users, and 32% for homosexual men. These findings have profound implications for multiprofessional working and the delivery of quality care.

Most importantly, these and other studies have set the agenda for the nursing response in the first decade of the AIDS pandemic. The nurse with experience in HIV and AIDS has so many unique contributions to make in so many other areas of nursing practice and in so many health-care settings. We currently live in a culture in which all too often the care and commitment of nurses is undervalued, as it is not easy to quantify. No patients have ever needed that care and commitment more than those with AIDS and HIV, and the need to base interventions on sound research information remains crucial. The relationship between research, practice, education and policy is currently being made increasingly clear by the development and dissemination plans of the Department of Health research strategy.

Research has already made a vital contribution to the provision of education and care in HIV and AIDS, and it is to be hoped that it remains a priority for the future.

REFERENCES

Akinsanya, J.A. and Rouse, P. (1991) *Who Will Care? A Survey of the Knowledge and Attitudes of Hospital Nurses to People With HIV/AIDS.* Report to the Department of Health, Anglia Polytechnic University.

Allen, I. and Hogg, D. (1993) *Work Roles and Responsibilities in Genitourinary Medicine Clinics*, Policy Studies Institute, London.

Bond, S. and Rhodes, T. (1990) HIV infection and community midwives: experience and practice. *Midwifery*, 6, 33–40, 86–92.

Bond, S., Rhodes, T., Philips, P. *et al.* (1989a) *A National Study of HIV Infection, AIDS and Community Nursing Staff.* Report to the Department of Health, Health Care Research Unit, University of Newcastle upon Tyne.

Bond, J., Bond, S., Donaldson, C. *et al.* (1989b) Training and Education in Response to HIV Infection: Surveys of General Practitioners and Community Nursing Staff, In *DH Yearbook of Research and Development*, HMSO.

Brown-Peterside, P., Sibbald, B. and Freeling, P. (1991) AIDS: knowledge, skills and attitudes among vocational trainees and their trainers. *British Journal of General Practice*, 41, 401–405.

Butterworth, C.A., Faugier, J. and Brocklehurst, (1993) *AIDS and Community Care. Discharge, Referral Patterns and Coordination.* School of Nursing Studies, The University of Manchester.

Faugier, J., Hayes, C. and Butterworth, C.A. (1992) *Drug Using Prostitutes: Their Health Care Needs and Their Clients.* Report to the Department of Health, University of Manchester Press, Manchester.

Gallagher, M., Rhodes, T., Foy, C. *et al.* (1989) *A National Study of HIV Infection, AIDS and General Practice*. Report to the Department of Health. Health Care Research Unit, University of Newcastle upon Tyne.

Glanz, A., Byrne, C. and Jackson, P. (1990) *Prevention of AIDS Among Drug Misusers. The Role of the High Street Pharmacy. Findings of a survey of community pharmacies in England and Wales*. Report to the Department of Health. Institute of Psychiatry, Addiction Research Unit, London.

McCann, K. and Wadsworth, E. (1991) The experience of having a positive HIV antibody test. *AIDS Care*, 3(1), 43–53.

McCann, K. and Wadsworth, E. (1992) The role of informal carers in supporting gay men who have HIV related illness: what do they do and what are their needs? *AIDS Care*, 4(1), 25–34.

Robinson, D., Maynard, A. and Tolley, K. (1991a) *HIV-AIDS and Social Care*. Discussion paper 81. Centre for Health Economics, University of York.

Robinson, D., Maynard, A. and Tolley, K. (1991b) HIV-AIDS Needs and Government Funding for Health and Social Care, in *Hospital Management International* (ed. L. Paine). Sterling Publications, London.

Robottom, B.M. (1989) *Managing the Nursing Care of People With AIDS in the Community – an Evaluation of Workshops*. Report to the Department of Health. The English National Board for Nursing, Midwifery and Health Visiting, London.

Sibbald, B., Freeling, H., Coles, H. and Wilkins, J. (1991) HIV/AIDS Workshop for primary health care staff. *Medical Education*, **25**, 243–250.

Stimson, G.V., Alldritt, L., Dolan, K. and Donoghue, M.C. (1989) Preventing the spread of HIV in injecting drug users, in *Proceedings of the 50th Annual Scientific Meeting of the Committee on Problems of Drug Dependence*, (ed. L.S. Harris), Monograph Series, National Institute of Drug Abuse, pp. 302–310, Carfax, Oxford.

UKCC for Nursing, Midwifery and Health Visiting (1990) *Report of Post Registration Education and Practice Project*, UKCC, London.

Wadsworth, E. and McCann, K. (1992) Attitudes towards and use of general practitioner services among homosexual men with HIV infection or AIDS. *British Journal of General Practice*, **42**, 107–110.

Clinical supervision and staff support in HIV and AIDS nursing

3

Jean Faugier and Ian Hicken

INTRODUCTION

The first 10 years of the AIDS pandemic has seen nurses and other health-care workers attempting to meet demands made on them in a climate in which organized staff support or clinical supervision was the exception rather than the norm. Things have recently changed dramatically with the policy statement of the Chief Nursing Officer, Mrs Yvonne Moores (1993), which calls for the rapid development and expansion of clinical supervision in all branches of nursing. Recent studies have demonstrated just how essential clinical supervision is for nurses working in this field, particularly for those coming into contact with HIV and AIDS for the first time.

Van Servellan *et al.* (1987), in a survey of nurses, found that fear of contagion and discomfort at caring for homosexual men was still present even following educational interventions. Wallack (1989) reported that 53% of staff surveyed admitted to sometimes avoiding procedures involving people with AIDS based on complex reasons, many of which they had never discussed with others. Other studies, such as those by Kelly *et al.* (1988) and Knox and Dow (1989), found that working with the terminally ill and a high prevalence of bias towards the gay lifestyle were major determinants of deficient care delivered to those with AIDS.

A burgeoning literature is making it increasingly clear that many nurses and other health professionals, while displaying an increased knowledge and benefiting from a number of educational initiatives, still retain concerns about contagion, homosexuality, drug misuse and the whole aspect of the care and treatment of people terminally ill with what is essentially a sexually transmissible disease (Barrick, 1988; Imperato *et al.*, 1988; Gallop *et al.*, 1988).

AIDS and HIV, while often providing models of good practice in a wide variety of practical and psychological approaches to care, also have the ability to expose the fears, prejudices and concerns of professionals and their need for effective support and supervision.

Literature describing the implementation and practice of clinical supervision is fairly easy to find when it relates to professions such as psychotherapy, counselling and social work. However, until recently, little of any substance had been published in the nursing literature, and the absence of empirical data on clinical supervision remains widespread in all fields, particularly in nursing: in a majority of cases the term 'clinical supervision' has found its way into the vocabulary of AIDS and HIV nursing and, unlike other branches of nursing, has to some small extent had an impact on the nature of education and practice.

In cases, the word supervision is automatically associated with a management relationship. Indeed, it is suggested by Hill (1989) that people at work tend to think of their supervisors as authoritarian and that the whole concept of supervision is linked conceptually to an authority figure. Watt (1987) states that: 'the generally held conception of supervision is of a lower management activity in which a group of workers is overseen by a supervisor for a variety of reasons such as ensuring timekeeping, processing pay entitlements, regulating rates of work, and monitoring the quality of work according to pre-set standards. Literature from North America continues this theme, pointing to what is claimed to be a distinct difference in the understanding of clinical supervision between nurses and other disciplines involved in therapeutic input, especially in psychiatry'. 'Many nurses have misconceptions about the nature of clinical supervision. They may be depriving themselves of one of the most valuable tools in existence for learning and refining skills of assessment and treatment of patients' (Platt-Koch, 1986). In a full description of the use of clinical supervision, Platt-Koch also points to the lack of clear understanding of the nature of clinical supervision among nurses: 'To many nurses, supervision means observation by an administrative superior who inspects, directs, controls and evaluates the nurse's work'.

Work in the area of child protection found that a key issue in contributing to the development of nursing practice was the separation of managerial and clinical supervisory roles into twin spheres and between different individuals. This increased the managers' ability to manage and provided staff with supervisors with up-to-date skills who possessed credibility in a difficult area of nursing practice.

The other assumption most common in nursing stems from a view of clinical supervision simply as a provision of support for a nursing workforce suffering from stress or in danger of 'burnout'. This misunderstanding is typified by the all too frequent belief that clinical supervision can be equated to an informal peer support group, the 'tea break/tear break', as described by Butterworth and Faugier (1992). This is not to say, however, that such informal support is not an important safety valve, particularly in the absence of any more formalized systems of supervision.

Until recently, very few models of clinical supervision were formalized at an organizational level. Such models have existed for some time in mental health nursing, and more frequently in specialist settings, often based on a therapeutic community approach: thus, in some of the larger institutions and inpatient settings, group supervision was an approach sometimes found to be an integral part of nursing practice on more progressive wards and units. Clinical supervision in these settings was frequently delivered by nurses who had undergone training in other therapeutic approaches, often practitioners with backgrounds in psychodynamic therapy. In this sense, supervision was not seen as the right and responsibility of every mental health nurse, as Ivey (1977) pointed out: 'Supervision in the helping professions has too long been reserved for the master practitioner'. Additionally, such supervision was more frequently aimed at the therapeutic 'milieu' and the nursing relationship with groups rather than the clinical supervision of individualized nursing care.

Extended clinical practice, greater autonomous practice and a greater degree of responsibility for decision making have combined to increase awareness of the need for clinical supervision. In addition, the recent development of the internal market in the NHS and the changes in community care management brought about by the Community Care Act (1993), combined with the implications of the Children's Act (1992), have all added to the demands on expertise felt by mental health nursing practitioners (Laurent, 1993). While some nurses do undoubtedly take the initiative and make their own arrangements for clinical supervision, either as individuals, ward teams or community peer groups, it is interesting to note that, as Butterworth and Faugier (1992) point out, the strategies many nurses use to deal with the demands of clinical nursing and its inherent interpersonal relationship issues are not always enabling, and frequently remain ill defined. Increasing numbers of nurses have found that the supervisory process, properly and responsibly facilitated, can, as Critchley (1987) indicates, assist in the refinement of their abilities to observe more precisely, to understand and describe more accurately, and to assume less about their own and their clients' behaviours and needs.

Platt-Koch (1986) advocates regular formalized clinical supervision as the major method of learning and refining skills: 'One cannot learn how to interact therapeutically with a patient solely by reading a book. The nurse needs to practise therapeutic skills, have successes and failures, and learn from the inevitable mistakes. The key to learning is for the nurse to review the work with a senior clinician, one with more experience and enough skill to facilitate objective self-evaluation by the nurse. Through this process of clinical supervision the nurse's strengths are acknowledged and professional weakness or learning needs are identified.' Stating that undertaking nursing without adequate clinical supervision constitutes a disservice to the patient, Platt-Koch (1986) makes a similar point as Casement (1985), in noting that even the most seasoned professional will retain 'psychological blind spots' and need the relationship of supervision to fully understand the nature of interactions with patients. Casement (1985), while advocating the development of 'the internal supervisor', which involves the very high-level skill of examining one's own interactions and understandings critically and dynamically, also maintains that this can only be achieved with regular high-quality external supervision. Similarly, Sundeen *et al.* (1985) argue that the need for supervision is never lost, regardless of the amount of experience a nurse may have.

DEFINITION OF TERMS

Mentorship and preceptorship schemes have developed momentum over the past decade and are particularly associated with nurse education, and more specifically with Project 2000. The major objective of such schemes is to provide the support and educational input in the practice setting which was widely viewed as fundamental to the development and success of Project 2000.

Darling (1984), a pioneer of mentorship in the United States, has outlined what she perceives as the characteristics of 'good mentors'. These include the following roles:

- an envisioner: giving the learner a picture of what nursing can be like;
- a standard prodder: pushing the learner to achieve high standards;
- a challenger: making the learner look more closely at her skills and the decisions she makes.

Also emphasizing the educational aspects of 'mentorship', Puetz (1985) describes mentors as enhancing their protégés' skills and furthering their intellectual ability. The majority of nurse educators in the United Kingdom, having become deskilled through a lack of consistent practice, would not be able to fit this definition and therefore cannot be seen as adequate mentors. Other writers, such as Burnard (1989), claim that if students are exposed to the skills involved in positive mentorship, especially active listening and empathy, they will be more inclined to employ similar therapeutic exchanges with patients. It remains the case, however, that in the majority of schemes mentorship is linked to academic achievement and success rather than the refinement of skill and the improvement of care.

Preceptorship is presented as a self-limited relationship aimed at facilitating the transition from student to newly qualified and confident practitioner. In many ways, the model postulated by the majority of writers closely resembles that employed in educational settings, where newly qualified teachers are required to serve a probationary period before being accepted as a fully fledged practitioner. Much of the research work available in this field is American; it is therefore difficult to draw many lessons from its results which may be globally applicable to the situation in the United Kingdom. However, some studies – Myrick and Awrey (1988); Foy and Waltho (1991) – conclude that, overall, preceptorship is a positive assistance in enabling students to move more readily into their new role as qualified practitioners.

In the field of counselling, and this is of course particularly relevant in HIV and AIDS care, there has been an increasing emphasis on supervision, which must ultimately influence client care rather than result in supervisees becoming more aware of their own psychological problems. In arguing that supervision in counselling should be mandatory and non-negotiable, Proctor (1991) makes the case that: 'supervision is non-negotiable because the aim at its simplest is to equip practitioners to use counselling interactions skilfully and appropriately in their working situations. Personal supervision is the opportunity to share working practice in detail. Here it is possible to develop the ability to monitor one's work'. Other areas of supervision seen as vitally important in counselling are the receipt of direct personal feedback, the supply of appropriate guidance and information from a more experienced practitioner, and the provision of a safe and challenging forum in which to examine issues of outcome and professional accountability.

Research into the effectiveness of supervision programmes in other disciplines – mainly counselling, psychotherapy and psychology – has concentrated on attempting to evaluate the developmental models of supervision most frequently utilized in the United States. This research, by Stoltenburg and Delworth (1987) and Holloway (1984) puts forward a tentative model by which it is possible to examine the various interactions/transactions of the supervisory relationship and its consequent impact on the supervisee. Although research in this area is very difficult, time consuming and open to the usual criticisms levelled at process research, there is nevertheless a need to develop models capable of determining the factors which are prerequisites for clinical supervision as well as the various behaviour stages that supervisors and supervisees are likely to encounter. This would provide a stimulation and a guide to those undertaking further much-needed research.

In another, earlier, attempt to categorize the roles of the clinical supervisor, Frankham (1987) offered the 'twelve-role model of supervisor functions'. In an examination of this model, Simms (1993) has superimposed Proctor's 'three function model' of supervision in order to draw out the primary aim of each role. For the purpose of this chapter, Frankham's model has been altered to address AIDS and HIV issues more directly:

- Monitor: to ensure the maintenance of professional standards (**normative**);
- Manager: to ensure the pursuit of agency practice and policy. This is particularly important in relation to prejudice, equity and confidentiality (**normative**);
- Teacher: to impart nursing theory and knowledge in an attempt to challenge attitudes (**formative**);
- Mentor: to provide a supportive and sustaining relationship (**restorative**);
- Therapist: to provide counselling or therapy aimed at providing patients with the means to change high-risk behaviour in the interests of themselves and the rest of society, and to come to terms with their own position (**restorative**);
- Analyst: to provide insights into the process of nursing and the elements of the supervisory relationship (**formative**);
- Mirror: to facilitate the supervisee's explorations (**restorative/ formative**);
- Trainer: to provide training in practical nursing skills (**formative**);
- Evaluator: to assess nursing competence and standards of individualized nursing care (**normative/formative**);
- Reviewer: to formulate and review nursing care plans, intervention and outcomes together with the supervisee (**normative/formative**);

- Facilitator: to assess the supervisee's levels of stress and establish support needs (**restorative**);
- Professional representative: to provide a role model of professional practice (**formative/normative**).

Those models that have had perhaps the most significant impact on supervision and its practice in a number of disciplines are those coming under the broad umbrella of 'developmental models'. These models have their roots very firmly in clinical supervision in psychoanalysis, and are currently widely practised by those who supervise psychotherapists and counsellors. However, they also have much to offer to practitioners in the AIDS field, who operate through relatively in-depth case work. As such, these models are easily adaptable to the community setting, where nurses working in HIV and AIDS are frequently involved in such relationships with clients, and to the key worker/named nurse situations pertaining in many inpatient settings.

The two-matrix model divides supervision into two main categories:

- supervision which directly focuses on the treatment/care matrix, in which supervisee and supervisor reflect together on observed practice, reports, written notes or recordings of the nurse client interaction;
- supervision which focuses on the treatment/care matrix through its reflection in the 'here and now' experience of the supervision process.

These can be further subdivided into two approaches which will guide the supervision session:

- Approach 1: AIDS/HIV nursing practice is reported and reflected on in the supervision session: this is done in three stages:

  1. Reflection on the content of nursing practice: Attention here is focused on the client, the client's life, what he/she has been able to share or explore with the nurse, which area of his/her life, which health or other problem is currently in need of change or attention. This form of clinical supervision focuses on the relationship between client needs and the process of nursing.

  2. Exploration of the strategies and interventions used by the nurse to meet the client's needs: The focus here is on the choices used by the nurse: not only what interventions were used but also when and why they were used. Alternative strategies and interventions might be developed and their consequences anticipated. The main goal of this form of supervision would be to increase the nurse's choices and skills in intervention.

3.   Exploration of the nursing process and relationship: Here, the supervisor will pay particular attention to what was happening, consciously or unconsciously, in the process of delivery of nursing care. Hawkins and Shohet (1989) refer to this as examining 'what happens around the edges': the metaphors and images, the worries and concerns of nurses about clients which may provide essential insights into vitally important issues for the maintenance of high standards of care.

- Approach 2: Focus on the nursing process as it is reflected in the supervisory process; this is also done in three stages:

1.   Focus on the nurse's countertransference: This is an extremely important aspect of nursing practice, and supervision should improve awareness of the influence of such dynamic material on practice and relationships. Here, the supervisor concentrates on whatever is still being carried by the nurse from the process of nursing the client. The countertransference may be of three different kinds: personal material from the nurse which has been restimulated by the process of nursing a particular client; the nurse's unconscious attempt to 'counter' the transference of the client; and projected material from the client that the nurse has 'taken in' somatically, physically or mentally (Casement, 1985; Hobson, 1985).

2.   Focus on the here-and-now process as a mirror of the there-and-then process: Here, the supervisor focuses on the relationship in the supervision session in order to explore how it might be unconsciously playing out or paralleling the hidden dynamics of the relationship with the client. Difficulties in the relationship between therapist and patient are reflected in the relationship difficulties between therapist and supervisor. Eckstein and Wallenstein (1958) described what they termed the 'parallel process', which they observed more frequently in inexperienced therapists. This process frequently arises when the nurse – and this is particularly pertinent to HIV and issues of sexuality – responds to those aspects of the patient's problems that highlight her own personal learning blocks as they are activated by the supervisory relationship.

3.   Focus on the supervisor's countertransference: Here the supervisor primarily focuses on his/her own 'here-and-now' experience in supervision and on the feelings, thoughts and images which the shared material or discussion gives rise to. These insights can be used to provide reflective illumination for the nurse in supervision and assists the process of working on two levels, because the material which has been unheard at a conscious level may emerge in the supervisor's thoughts, feelings and images of the

supervisory process. However, some of this material may need to be retained and remain unshared with the supervisee, and may be more properly dealt with in the supervisor's own supervision.

GROUP SUPERVISION

With a workforce of the size and complexity of nursing, individual clinical supervision on a regular basis may be impossible. In some situations where there is a definite team nursing approach, it may also be inappropriate. On the other hand, the potential for group supervision in this and other branches of nursing remains enormous. However, the distinction must be made between group supervision, which is a formalized regular meeting in a setting covered by agreed ground rules on issues such as respect and confidentiality, and an informal peer-group meeting, which is simply a coming together of colleagues, usually for support at a particularly stressful time.

Taerk *et al.* (1993) describe work using group methods of supervision and training with health-care professionals, many of whom were nurses. Although this work was essentially a research study and was therefore time limited, it provides real insights into the use of groups in dealing with the 'big issues' in HIV, namely fear of contagion, homophobia and prejudice as to the lifestyles of others, and fears of feelings of attachment and loss. The groups provided an opportunity to discuss feelings and concerns, and express conflicts. The group leader's role was to encourage expression, confirm reality and facilitate acceptance of conflicting feelings in health-care workers.

The selection and convening of groups for supervision needs time and consideration. Ideally, a group should be facilitated by a leader who is more experienced and skilled than the group members, and who has access to regular support and supervision. However, if set up properly and supported adequately, peer-group supervision can be a useful means of improving practice in mental health nursing, particularly if a few ground rules are observed:

- The group should have shared values but contain within it experience of differing approaches and therapeutic skills, to avoid collusion and lowering of horizons.
- A group should ideally contain no more than seven people: supervision needs time, and if the group is to meet the needs of its members it must be limited in size.
- The group should have a clear commitment from all its members. Resistance to supervision needs to be examined and used as a learning experience.

- The group should operate on the basis of a clearly established contract covering aspects of time, place, frequency, duration, confidentiality and boundaries.
- Groups must be clear about their focus. It is useful to attempt to ascertain members' expectations and agendas.
- There must be clearly defined roles within the group, in order to determine which member is going to be responsible for the organization, who carries the main responsibility for facilitating and for managing time and interruptions.
- The group must plan regular review sessions and the regular input of external supervisors who can look at the work from different angles.
- In AIDS and HIV it is possible that the group may also need to deal with the issue of ill and infected group members, and this needs to be clearly addressed and acknowledged and issues of confidentiality examined.

However, it must be remembered that groups may also present a number of pitfalls and, in the wrong hands, can be extremely destructive (Wright, 1989). Consequently, any service wishing to establish a network of peer-group clinical supervision should invest first in training for group leadership to ensure that nurses have some idea of the power of group dynamics.

Of similar importance in terms of investment is the development of senior clinical nurses who will act as the 'culture carriers' of nursing. This key link individual in relation to both research and practice is in a pivotal position to ensure the right atmosphere for learning and research (Pembry, 1980; Ogier, 1982). More recently, however, the senior clinical nurse has been increasingly described as someone responsible for guiding the actions of others rather than providing direct patient care.

There is now a wealth of documentation on the central position occupied by senior clinical nurses or clinical nurse specialists in providing support to learners in the clinical environment, and on the subsequent benefits this has for improved practice (Booth, 1992; Sloan and Slevin, 1991; Clifford, 1992). However, many studies have demonstrated that senior nurses themselves, the very people expected to provide a positive supportive learning environment, have their own very real needs for support and will be unable to respond to requests for cooperation with educational and research initiatives without it (Cooper, 1988; Mackay, 1989; Hingley and Harris, 1986). Many nurses working in a senior position in the AIDS field who are suitable candidates for the role of clinical supervisor to more junior staff, may feel threatened by change and simply develop a system which is unstructured and which exists largely on paper. The responsibilities facing a professional supervisor are onerous: nurses undertaking such work need to be sure that the advice and information they are giving is up to date, professional and research based. One can easily imagine how some senior nurses who have lost touch with practice will attempt to avoid this relationship. As Hawkins and Shohet (1989) have said: 'It is easier to use less structured types of supervision to avoid the rigours and concentrated focus of regular, formal sessions....It is easy to create a climate where supervision is only requested when you have a recognizable problem and at other times you have to be seen to soldier on'.

TRAINING AND PREPARATION OF CLINICAL SUPERVISORS

Mental health nurses who practise as clinical supervisors usually tend to supervise in the manner in which they themselves were supervised (Clarkson and Gilbert, 1991). Therefore, training nurses to become more conscious of their roles as clinical supervisors may involve some 'unlearning' to ensure that they concentrate on clinical nursing and are not tempted to lead their supervisees only towards their own therapeutic approach.

Authors such as Robinson (1974) and Clarkson and Gilbert (1991) have suggested a structured approach to the preparation of supervisors using models that propose a period of supervised practice. This implies that the trainee supervisor who is working with more senior trainers will also deliver supervision to less experienced nursing staff. According to this approach, there should be three structured stages of training:

- Awareness: bringing the supervisor from unconscious incompetence to conscious incompetence.
- Accommodation: making the move from conscious incompetence to conscious competence.
- Assimilation: from conscious to unconscious competence.

In order to facilitate this process, the training of supervisors will need to address the extent of the senior nurse's knowledge base, as an expert command of the subject area is a prerequisite for quality supervision. 'Any trainer requires a firm grasp of the material, sufficient experience to provide a fertile source for examples, and an ongoing sensitivity to the vicissitudes of practice. Supervising clinicians who remain in the field, working with the ongoing challenges of their practice, are usually experienced as having greater authority and authenticity as trainers than supervisors who are no longer active in clinical practice' (Clarkson and Gilbert, 1991).

Research into AIDS and HIV nursing has been aware of the role nurse educators could potentially play in clinical supervision, and contains recommendations requiring them to continue to practise as do our medical and psychological colleagues in teaching positions (Bond, ; Akinsanya, ; Butterworth and Faugier *et al.*,).

Nurses in this field are subject to the common mental blocks to further learning that affect the general population. This, combined with the culture of nursing, which has tended to view qualification as a certificate of continuing competence, produces a challenging climate for the introduction of clinical supervision.

Experience as a practitioner and supervisor of nurses in primary health care has shown how relevant is the comparison made by Hawkins and Shohet (1991) between clinical supervision and what the British coalminers used to call 'pit-head time', i.e. the right to wash off the grime of the job in the bosses' time. Clinical supervision is 'pit-head time' for those who work at the coalface of emotional distress, disease, loss, death and confusion. Nurses working in AIDS and HIV work at one of the most distressing and challenging coalfaces on which any professional could be employed, and their need for effective clinical supervision is unquestionable. A major theme of the literature on nursing and AIDS has been that nurses and other health-care workers display 'bad attitudes' and that these attitudes often lead to inferior care. The answer in most parts of the country has been to increase educational initiatives which, it is hoped, will change attitudes and therefore improve the quality of care. Although there is evidence that some of these educational initiatives have had the desired effect of changing 'expressed' attitudes, there is little evidence that they have had the effect of convincing staff that their concerns are being treated legitimately. On the contrary, some educational programmes simply teach health-care staff that their attitudes are not acceptable and should not be expressed, thereby causing resentment and driving the expression of such attitudes to a deeper, less conscious level, which is much more dangerous to the delivery of effective and appropriate care.

Recent work with community nurses (Butterworth *et al.*, 1993) has confirmed the claim by Taerk *et al.* (1993) that nursing staff have a strong desire to help patients and often experience shame at their inability to feel empathic towards those with AIDS. Often they display this by poor boundary management and a need to do more to counter their negative feelings. Effective clinical supervision can assist nurses to channel this energy and commitment in the best interests of the client and their own self-esteem.

REFERENCES

Barrick, B. (1988) The willingness of nursing personnel to care for patients with acquired immune deficiency syndrome: a survey study and recommendations. *Journal of Professional Nursing*, **4**, 366–72.

Booth, K. (1992) Providing support and reducing stress, in *Clinical Supervision and Mentorship in Nursing*, (eds C. A. Butterworth and J. Faugier), Chapman & Hall, London, pp. 50–9.

Burnard, P. (1989) The role of the mentor. *Journal of District Nursing*, **8**(3), 8–17.

Butterworth, C.A. and Faugier, J (eds) (1992) *Clinical Supervision and Mentorship in Nursing*, Chapman & Hall, London.

Casement, P. (1985) *On Learning from the Patient*, Tavistock, London.

Clarkson, P. and Gilbert, M. (1991) The training of counsellor trainers and supervisors, in *Training and Supervision for Counselling in Action*, (eds W. Dryden and B. Thorne), Sage Publications, London, pp. 143–70.

Clifford, C. (1992) *The Clinical Role of the Nurse Teacher*. Paper presented to the Royal College of Nursing Research Advisory Group Annual Conference, University of Birmingham, April 1992.

Cooper, C. (1988) Stress, Mental Health and Job Satisfaction. *Health Services Management Research*, 1.1.

Critchley, D.L. (1987) Clinical supervision as a learning tool for the therapist in milieu settings. *Journal of Psychological Nursing*, **25**(8).

Darling, L.A. (1984) What do nurses want in a mentor? *Journal of Nursing Adminstration*, **14**(10), 42–4.

Eckstein, R. and Wallenstein, R.S. (1958) *The Teaching and Learning of Psychotherapy*, Basic Books, New York.

Faugier, J (1992) The supervisory relationship, in *Clinical Supervision and Mentorship in Nursing*, (eds C. A. Butterworth and J. Faugier).

Foy, H. and Waltho, B.J. (1991) The mentor system: are learner nurses benefiting? *Senior Nurse*, **9**(5), 24–5.

Frankham, H. (1987) *Aspects of Supervision, Counsellor Satisfaction, Utility and Defensiveness and Tasks in Supervision*, Dissertation, Roehampton Institute of the University of Surrey.

Gallop, R.M., Taerk, G., Lancee, W.J. *et al.* (1988) *Acceptable Risk*, Cambridge University Press.

Hawkins, P. and Shohet, R. (1989) Approaches to the supervision of counsellors: the supervisory relationship, in *Training and Supervision for Counselling in Action*, (eds W. Dryden and B. Thorne), Sage, London, pp. 99–116.

Hill, J. (1989) Supervision in the caring professions: a literature review. *Community Psychiatric Nursing Journal*, **9**(5), 9–15.

Hingley, P. and Harris, P. (1986) Burnout at Senior Level, *Nursing Times*, **86**(31), 28–9.

Hobson, R. (1985) *Forms of Feeling: The Heart of Psychotherapy*. Tavistock, London.

Holloway, E.L. (1984) Outcome evaluation in supervision research. *Counselling Psychologist (USA)*, **12**(3), 167–74.

Imperato, P.J., Fieldman, J.G., Nayeri, K. and Dehovitz, J.A. (1988) Medical students' attitudes towards caring for patients with AIDS in a high incidence area. *New York State Journal of Medicine*, **88**, 223–7.

Ivey, A. (1977) Foreword, in *Supervision of Allied Training. A Comparative Review*, (eds D. J. Kurpius, R.D. Baker and I.D. Thomas), Greenwood Press, London.

Kelly, J.A., St-Lawrence, J.S., Hood, H.V. *et al.* (1988) Nurses' attitudes towards AIDS. *Journal of Continuing Education for Nurses*, **19**(2), 78–83.

Knox, M.D. and Dow, M.G. (1989) *Staff discomfort in working with HIV spectrum patients.* V International Conference on AIDS: The Scientific and Social Challenge, Montreal. Abstract MDP60.

Laurent, C. (1993) Out in force. *Nursing Times*, **89**(3),

Mackay, L. (1989) *Nursing a problem*, Open University Press, Milton Keynes.

Moores, Y. (1993) *Vision for the future – a strategy for nursing*, Department of Health, HMSO.

Myrick, F. and Awrey, J. (1988) The effect of preceptorship on the clinical competency of baccalaureate student nurses: a pilot study. *Canadian Journal of Nursing Research*, **20**(3), 29–43.

Ogier, M.E. (1982) *An Ideal Sister?* RCN, London.

Pembrey, S. (1980) *The Ward Sister, Key to Nursing*, RCN Publications, London.

Platt-Koch, L.M (1986) Clinical supervision for psychiatric nurses. *Journal of Psychological Nursing*, **26**(1), 7–15.

Proctor, B. (undated) Supervision: A cooperative exercise in accountability, in *Enabling and Ensuring*, (eds M. Marken and M. Payne). Leicester National Youth Bureau and Council for Education and Training in Youth and Community Work.

Proctor, B. (1991) On being a trainer, in *Training and Supervision for Counselling in Action*, (eds W. Dryden and B. Thorne), Sage, London, pp. 49–74.

Puetz, B.E. (1985) Learn the ropes from a mentor. *Nursing Success Today*, **2**(6), 11–13.

Simms, J. (1993) Supervision, in *Mental Health Nursing*, (eds H. Wright and M. Giddey), Chapman & Hall, London, pp. 328–44.

Sloan, P. and Slevin, D. (1991) *Teaching and Supervision of Student Nurses During Practice Placements*. Discussion paper [OP/NB/2/91] for the National Board for Nursing, Midwifery and Health Visiting for Northern Ireland, Belfast.

Stoltenberg, C.D. and Delworth, U. (1987) *Supervising Counsellors and Therapists*, Jossey Bass, San Francisco.

Sundeen, S.J., Stuart, G.W., Rankin, E.D. and Cohen, S.A. (1985) *Nurse–Client Interaction*. Mosby, St Louis.

Van Servellen, G.M., Lewis, C.E. and Leake, B. (1987) How nurses feel about AIDS. *Nursing*, **17**, 8.

Wallack, J.J. (1989) AIDS anxiety among health care professionals. *Hospital and Community Psychiatry*, **40**, 507–10.

Watt, G. (1987) *Clinical Supervision in Community Psychiatric Nursing*. Unpublished report, Leeds University.

Wright, H. (1989) *Groupwork: Perspectives and Practice*, Scutari Press, Oxford.

AIDS: ethical dilemmas and the nursing response 4

Steve Wright

'And every day more crazies who debate
with phantom enemies on the street'
Thom Gunn, *An Invitation* 1992

INTRODUCTION

As the implications of HIV and AIDS began to sink into the collective consciousness of nursing in the 1980s, the response at one level was at first fairly pragmatic. The greater part of the nursing literature at that time focused very much on matters of infection control, protecting immunosuppressed patients, dealing with chemotherapy and so on. In fact, the emphasis was very much on managing the 'illness' almost as if it were a separate entity from the person. Frank (1991) argues that such a response is typical of health-care professionals, who seek to 'manage' a health problem as if it were a disease 'out there', divorced from the human body, identifiable, containable, controllable, almost as if it were an entity unto itself. Faced with the myths and mysteries of HIV and AIDS at that time, the tendency to cling to tried and trusted aspects of disease control perhaps served to allay anxiety among nurses about their ability to cope. Protected by the safety of set rules and procedures, anxieties can be contained using these old patterns (Menzies, 1961).

Paradoxically, it was nurses who also proved to be at the leading edge of care. In contrast to many individuals and groups of other professions, many nurses were at the forefront of innovative practice, determining new care needs and setting up new services, fighting bigotry and ignorance with what could sometimes be described as heroism in the face of ignorance and prejudice throughout society. HIV has presented a great challenge to nurses, confronting as it does their values, practices and prejudices and many ethical dilemmas concerning autonomy, control and confidentiality. The emergence of HIV has tested to the limits the ability of nurses to give compassionate non-judgemental care. Many nurses have risen positively to this challenge, but it has also brought real dilemmas to many.

For most nurses, HIV and AIDS remained something of a (frightening) mystery, whipped up by the hysteria of the popular press and out of proportion to the then actual numbers of affected people in the UK. Indeed, as 1993 drew to a close, the RCN found itself castigated in the press for 'scaremongering' in the early 1980s, when it predicted, along with many others, that a million people would be HIV positive within 10 years (RCN, 1985). The reality was indeed far removed from this. A written House of Commons reply indicated that up to 31 March 1993 there were 7341 reported cases of AIDS in the UK and 19 524 people were reported HIV positive. From 1986 to 1993, the government had spent £105 million on AIDS research and £14 million centrally on public education about AIDS. From 1989 to 1992, a further £65 million was contributed to local prevention initiatives. These figures do not include much of the local and regional spending. The government spent more on public HIV education than on any other health promotion programme (Hansard, 1993).

Interestingly, the fact that the 'worst-case' scenarios had not emerged led not to recognition that existing health promotion strategies might be working and should be renewed and strengthened, but rather it was argued that resources could now be reduced, that many responsible bodies were 'wrong', or that the extent and dangers of HIV and AIDS had indeed been a myth promoted by various interested parties, such as some sectors of the medical research establishment, 'gay' lobbyists and so on (Connor, 1994; Illman, 1993).

The medical model provides a fairly pragmatic approach to dealing with a disease which in many respects is no more difficult to deal with than any other communicable disease (Patton, 1990). However, the disease orientation of the medical model often fails, as in this case, to take account of the patients' perceptions of their illness, of the values and beliefs of nurses who deliver care, or of the social context in which care is taking place. Thus the early advice available to nurses has been balanced in recent years by the recognition of the support needed by them and the profound ethical dilemmas they face. The practical aspects of caring for the patient with AIDS are relatively simple. However, AIDS is not a disease like any other, as some have claimed (Ingrams, 1990). The stigma and misconceptions, the prejudices acted out on those who are HIV positive, the financial and social implications – all these combine to create a health-care problem in which an exclusive focus on the disease process is woefully inadequate. How do patients feel, not only about the fear of death, but about how they will be treated by society once a diagnosis is made? How do nurses respond to their own values and prejudices? Nurses, after all, are part of society themselves, and subject to the effects of the same commonly held values, media exposure and socialization.

However, it is presumed that nurses, educated and aware of AIDS issues, will somehow respond differently from the general run of the population. For almost a decade the professional press has been deluged with papers on HIV and AIDS matters. Multitudes of books, videos, position papers, courses, support groups and so on have emerged. Professional advice, such as that produced by the UKCC, the RCN and the RCM has reiterated ethical principles of the nurse's duty to care, of safeguarding and promoting the interests and well-being of individual patients and clients, and of acting with 'beneficence', i.e. thinking and doing good.

The attention given to AIDS both professionally and publicly has led to some interesting dilemmas. Society has had to face up to its many inconsistencies and hypocrisies about sex. On the one hand prejudices and myths abound; on the other a plethora of AIDS-awareness approaches has multiplied in all avenues of the media. By the mid-1980s it became possible on the traditionally reticent, often prudish, British television, to have a young woman demonstrating the application of a condom to a model of an erect penis during a prime-time TV programme.

Nurses, like everyone else, have had to look at their own values and practices. The standards promoted by the professional and statutory organizations (UKCC, 1992a) tend to maintain the image of an army of compassionate and committed nurses who, it is assumed, will act responsibly, with up-to-date knowledge and practices, in the best interests of patients. The ideal appears somewhat different from the reality. Despite all the educational efforts, it seems that some nurses still leave much to be desired in their approach to the problems of AIDS. For example, more than two-thirds of nurses interviewed in a Department of Health-funded report on nursing and AIDS said that their colleagues were not adopting recommended infection control procedures for all patients (National Federation for Education Research, 1993).

The report also indicated that many took precautions only for patients known or suspected of being HIV positive. Some cited practical difficulties, such as emergencies and lack of access to supplies, and others disliked wearing gloves and other protective clothing. Although some nurses thought they were unlikely to encounter an HIV-positive patient in the near future, two-fifths were concerned about the possibility of contracting the disease from a patient. Such factors reinforce the view that there is a tension between the professional view of what nurses ought to know and how they should behave, and what nurses themselves feel able and willing to do. This is the territory of the ethical battleground for nurses. It is here that many of the most difficult and contentious aspects of caring for people who have AIDS or are HIV positive are found. Some of these issues, which have come to light in recent years, will be examined in more detail below.

NURSES AND THE DUTY TO CARE

There is a broad range of ethical and legal support for the view in the UK (UKCC, 1992a) that nurses should work with all patients, offering an equal standard of care regardless of factors such as age, religion, race, sexuality and so on. Nurses, therefore, have no rights to refuse to care for any patient, although they may, given certain provisions (e.g. prior notification to an employer), refuse to participate in abortion.

The ideal of nurses working to an equally high standard with all patients underpins the ethos of nursing worldwide. In practice, however, it is much more problematic and the issue of caring for people with HIV/AIDS has thrown the ideal/real contrast into sharp focus.

Some nurses clearly exhibit preferences for certain types of nursing (i.e. a particular specialty) and will tend to gravitate towards these. However, it becomes much more questionable if nurses choose a particular field of practice not on the basis of a particular interest but in order to avoid certain patients and their problems. It has already been suggested that despite their Code of Conduct (UKCC, 1992a), some nurses believe they can choose not to care for certain patients (Akinsanya and Rouse, 1992), most specifically patients with AIDS. Nurses seem able to use all kinds of tactics in order to avoid 'going public' over their preferences or prejudices, not least because of the strong generally accepted values within nursing that require nurses to think and behave in generally accepted ways. Any nurse who deviates from these views is likely to experience varying degrees of professional and public disapproval (Salvage, 1986), and may even find him or herself brought before an employer or the UKCC to face disciplinary action. The UKCC has the ultimate sanction of removing a nurse from the register (and hence denying them the title 'nurse' and the opportunity to practise as such).

Thus, it may be that nurses who feel prejudiced towards patients with AIDS will select areas of work where they feel they will be unlikely to encounter such people. This prejudice may be based on, for example, irrational fears of infection, or homophobia. This hidden iceberg of prejudice may only surface in collective surveys, such as the research by Akinsanya and Rouse (1992), or when individual nurses find themselves confronted with the reality of caring for a patient with AIDS.

Much early anecdotal evidence suggested that nurses made as many mistakes as others when they first encountered AIDS. Although many nurses approached this new health challenge positively, and shared the potential for nurses to be at the leading edge of humanitarian caring, others became bogged down by ignorance and prejudice. Excessive cross-infection measures, isolation of the patient, assumptions about patient lifestyles, failures in support and counselling – all of these and more have been raised as initial reactions by ignorant nurses to patients with AIDS. The setting up of specialist units and nursing roles, training courses, conferences, reports and so on has helped to diminish such problems by building awareness among nurses about the realities of AIDS. However, as the UKCC's recent development of the post-registration education concept (UKCC, 1993a) indicates, not all nurses are as adept at or committed to reading and studying widely in order to keep up to date. In addition, perceptions of AIDS based on prejudice and bigotry are unlikely to yield themselves to rational–empirical approaches. The notion that human beings will respond rationally by changing their behaviour when given clear knowledge and irrefutable evidence is not borne out by reality (Keyser, 1989). For example, smokers will not necessarily give up the habit despite being given the evidence of its dangers. Similarly, prejudices in nursing and negative values about certain patient groups or behaviours require much more imaginative approaches if they are to be changed.

Meanwhile, nurses have been given very clear messages in the UK that they cannot choose patients on the grounds of prejudice. In 1991, the first case in the UK occurred where a nurse was struck from the register for refusing to care for a patient with AIDS. The details of this particular incident are revealing. First, the nurse concerned appears to have been disciplined not so much because of her refusal to care but because she made a vociferous public display of it in the middle of the ward, causing distress to patients (UKCC, 1991). The manager also suggested that she would not have placed the nurse on that ward had she known in advance of her preferences. The inference to be drawn is that the issue would have been kept under wraps by a judicious placement of the nurse. The question of the acceptability of the nurse's prejudice appears to have been bypassed.

Conversely, it may well be that a patient with AIDS detects that a nurse assigned to his/her care is prejudiced, hostile or fails to meet his or her needs. Might the patient under these circumstances refuse care from a particular nurse?

Allowing patients and nurses to choose each other is fraught with moral and practical problems. The vast majority of nurses and patients do appear able to develop therapeutic relationships with each other. It is the nature of this relationship that is fundamental to healing.

Other authors have suggested that nurses who hold homophobic views and are reluctant to care for people with AIDS simply 'cannot be trusted' (Wells, 1988), while Pratt (1986) states firmly that those who discriminate by reluctance or refusal on any count should be counselled, given additional education and, if their reluctance persists, 'should be dismissed'.

Clearly, resorting immediately to disciplinary machinery, by either the employer or the professional body, is questionable if nurses have not themselves been given the opportunity to enhance their knowledge and skills. Many prejudices are based on ignorance of the facts. In addition, the preparation of nurses has traditionally given little attention to reflection and examination of their own attitudes, motives, values and fears. The provision for nurses to learn about themselves and change their behaviour is as important as, and a precursor to, Draconian disciplinary procedures. Even so, nurses who exhibit prejudiced behaviour not only raise questions about their own future in the profession, they also undermine professional credibility as a whole. 'A nursing service that includes discriminators who believe they can advocate, for example, for a white middle-class heterosexual, but who will not do the same for a gay man or i.v. drug user with or without AIDS, has to consider carefully the ethical issues of equity involved in claiming to be a service acting as the 'ideal' patient's advocate' (Mackereth, 1993).

TESTING OF HEALTH WORKERS

The risk of transmission of HIV from workers to patients is much lower than the risk faced by staff from infected patients. However, a scan through the British media in recent years reveals what seems at times to be an almost hysterical preoccupation with HIV-positive health workers – especially nurses and doctors. As a result, huge amounts of time and resources have been devoted by health organizations to tracing former patients of members of staff whose infection has become known. This knee-jerk response by health authorities has led many into extreme measures: setting up telephone helplines, mass contact tracing and calls for the mandatory testing of all health-care workers.

In the USA, in 1991, the Senate voted to impose prison sentences of at least 10 years and fines of up to $10,000 on health workers who have AIDS and who fail to tell patients on whom they have performed invasive procedures (BMJ, 1991).

A report of a BMA view (Hand, 1991) suggests that mandatory testing of all health workers is a waste of resources, but 'if you are a nurse or a doctor and you think you have been infected with HIV, then you have an ethical duty to be tested'. If the result of such a test is positive, Atkinson (1991) cautions nurses against declaring their status if the employer has no agreed methods of dealing with infected workers. The concerns of managers will tend to focus not only on the risks to patients, the exposure and subsequent 'bad press' if the case becomes publicly known, but also on the risk of employing someone who may have a long-term illness. At the same time, nurses and their managers are accountable for their actions. Practitioners who suspect they are infected should have the opportunity to be 'monitored regularly, and a positive test would mean ceasing to carry out functions that might put patients at risk'. In the case of midwives, for example, HIV infection would mean 'assessing their work and barring any risky procedures, such as suturing the perineum' (Hand, 1991).

When reports of HIV-positive health workers hit the headlines, the Royal College of Nursing AIDS Nursing Forum went on record as saying that it was 'alarmist to contact those people who were so unlikely to have been at risk'. In only one case in the USA (a dentist) has transmission from worker to patient been suggested. 'Given normal infection control procedures, there should be no reason to contact a patient simply because a health-care worker appears to be HIV positive. Only sexual or i.v. drug-using partners are at risk' (RCN, 1991). The UKCC supports this view and responded with the following guidance (UKCC, 1993c):

'Blood and body fluids from all patients pose a potential infection risk and appropriate precautions must be taken.

There is only one known authenticated instance of HIV transmission from an infected dentist to a patient. Safety comes through recognizing that all practitioners, like all patients, pose a potential infection risk, and all must ensure that high standards of clinical practice are maintained. The promotion of these standards is an important task for in-service education staff and for managers. Such standards require that, if a nurse, midwife or health visitor is infected with HIV, she or he take appropriate precautions to eliminate any possibility of blood or body fluid contamination to a patient. This necessitates the use of well established appropriate precautions to prevent transmission of any infection to a patient and, in some instances, reassignment of the practitioner to a different area of professional practice.

There have been a very limited number of documented incidents of HIV transmission by needlestick injuries, but the occupational risk of HIV transmission is minimal or even negligible if appropriate practice methods and strategies are diligently followed. These methods of reducing risk, appropriate to the setting, should be introduced and complied with. It must be emphasized, however, that such precautions amount to no more than the good clinical practice which all practitioners have a responsibility to maintain in all situations, irrespective of their serological status and any knowledge they may have of the serological status of their patients.'

The UKCC went on to oppose mandatory testing of health workers because it felt that such tests would 'generate a false sense of security' and risk lapses in hygiene standards if it was believed, falsely, that no HIV-positive practitioner was present. Furthermore, given the known seroconversion time (perhaps 3 months), even with frequent testing, there would be 'no guarantee that the practitioners involved in the care of patients are not infected'.

The same guidance from the UKCC reiterated the obligations of occupational health staff to maintain the confidentiality of staff who have sought testing. Each practitioner must be assessed on an individual basis and regularly. 'She or he must then act on the advice received' (UKCC, 1993c), as a result of which reassignment may be necessary to avoid procedures which may involve risks of transmission to patients.

The Department of Health (1991b) took a similar stance in its guidance, and recommended continuing education in this area, standards for infection control and health workers seeking advice if they know or suspect they are HIV positive. In the light of a crescendo of media reports in early 1993, the DoH (1993a) issued a press statement reaffirming its original guidance.

Interpretation of a clause in the original UKCC statement led some nurses to understand that 'if they believe or know' a colleague to be HIV positive, then they have a right to make such a matter known to an employer, or even the public. In a stormy debate at the RCN Congress in

1993 (RCN, 1993a) such 'unethical' behaviour was condemned. Anecdotes were given of nurses being reported to employers because they were thought to be gay or to take drugs (based on dubious interpretations of behaviour) and therefore 'believed' to be HIV positive. In the light of this furore, the UKCC agreed to revise its guidance and removed the offending section.

HIV TESTING AND SEROPREVALENCE

Initial arguments put forward for HIV testing were very seductive. In what was increasingly being seen as a crisis situation, mass screening of huge numbers of the public, through a variety of methods, appeared to be one way of tackling a major health menace. Many options were on offer and widely reported and advocated in the media, for example, testing all patients coming into hospital; all prisoners; visitors to the UK; children in school; and so on. Some of the discussion of this type around testing confirmed some of the worst fears of those working in the field and those who were at risk, namely, public and political talk of 'isolating' HIV carriers.

The stigmatizing effects of being HIV positive are profound and transcend those of any other disease. On the other hand, there was strong pressure for information on the extent to which HIV was spreading in the population, not least to determine appropriate health education approaches and future resources needed for care. One method advocated within the medical profession was to conduct trials anonymously. Selected groups of the population could be used to test for HIV at the same time as blood samples were taken for other reasons. The samples could be anonymized and in this way, it was argued, no test result could be traced back to an individual. This would give a picture of the spread of HIV while avoiding the disadvantages to the individual.

The Department of Health issued information on anonymous HIV testing in November 1988 (DoH, 1988). It based some of its views on the Cox report (DoH and Welsh Office, 1987) on the short-term prediction of HIV infection and AIDS in England and Wales, which explicitly recommended anonymous testing. The government saw no legal obstacles to such testing and no ethical objection to the testing, for scientific purposes, of blood samples taken properly in the first place for another purpose from a patient no longer identifiable. The Medical Research Council was therefore invited to bring forward proposals for a programme of anonymous screening within 3 months.

Early advice from the DoH suggested that there was no need to tell a patient, either individually or through public notices in a clinic, that his or her blood would be, or might be, anonymously tested. Provided the blood was to be used for the test for which it was given, and for which consent had been obtained, there was no bar to using any residue for other anonymous tests (DoH, 1988). However, what is lawful is not necessarily ethical, and in this case the legality of anonymous HIV testing without consent was questionable. Battery (deliberate touching of another without consent, or which is otherwise offensive or harmful) is unlawful. The tort of negligence means that the doctor and others have a legal duty to seek to ensure that the patient is appropriately informed of the relevant facts relating to a procedure, its purposes and the consequences for the patient of the procedure. Thus doctors, nurses and others are open to charges of assault and/or negligence when participating in HIV testing procedures without patient consent. Legal advice sought by the RCN at that time supported this view, as did a subsequent statement from the UKCC:

'On the specific issue of the taking of blood for testing without consent, the Council advises all its practitioners that they expose themselves to the possibility of civil action for damages, of criminal charges of assault or battery or of complaint to their regulatory body (the Council) alleging misconduct if they personally take the blood specimens, and of aiding and abetting an assault or battery if they cooperate in obtaining such specimens. The making of statements aimed at leading patients to believe that blood specimens taken for HIV testing were for some other purpose might also be construed as misconduct in a professional sense. In these respects blood taken for HIV testing is no different from blood samples are being taken for any laboratory examination' (UKCC, 1993b).

It has been argued that health professionals need not fear legal redress if they act in the interests of the greater public good (MRC, 1988; Emson, 1989). However, the law does not recognize any public policy justification that would render lawful the otherwise unlawful touching of the patient when the reason offered is for the benefit of others.

To allay some of the fears about testing, and in response to challenges to its policy, the DoH reviewed its plans and decided that testing should take place only on the basis of public awareness of the programme. This enabled the UKCC and the RCN, which had been monitoring the situation very closely, to update their guidance (UKCC, 1993b; RCN, 1992a). Provided certain conditions were met, the seroprevalence tests, with some reservations, could be supported if conducted in the agreed manner (UKCC, 1993a; RCN, 1992a). Provided there was public awareness of surveys, opportunities to opt out, and that staff were aware and able to inform patients, then the professional bodies felt able to support these initiatives.

In November 1989, the DoH put forward the following:

- A leaflet for patients informing them that anonymous testing is taking place, that they have a right not to take part and that their wishes will be respected, and advising them to ask the doctor, nurse or midwife if they have any questions.
- A poster in English and seven other languages making the same points.
- A leaflet for NHS staff providing details of the studies – why they are being done, how they will be done and additional information to enable them to answer patients' questions.
- A ministerial press conference announcing the studies and the publicity material.
- A briefing for staff at the national AIDS helpline to enable them to give advice in English and seven other languages to anyone worried about anonymous testing.
- A briefing for organizations such as the Health Education Authority, so that they can include information in any future educational material about HIV and AIDS.

Even so, reservations about the practicality of this approach persisted, as evidenced in statements made in the debate at the RCN congress of 1992. It remained clear that many nurses and patients were still unaware of the areas in which testing was taking place. This type of research therefore prompted many concerns:

- Testing patients without their explicit consent may undermine the essential trusting relationship between patient and carer. Without trust, the relationship cannot be therapeutic. Without trust, it is not possible to exercise the concept of partnership with the patient, which underpins therapeutic nursing activity. Many people have strong views about being involved and informed about actions that affect their bodies.
- Can anonymity be guaranteed? Technically this is possible, but uncertainties must arise, for example over the recent Scottish surveys where the marital status, week of birth and postcode were used to label the specimens. Could an unscrupulous person gain access to this information and use it to disadvantage the patient? Similar concerns about confidentiality have been raised over the

recently reported studies on pregnant African women at St Thomas' Hospital in London (de Selincourt 1992).

- How many patients might be discouraged from seeking help (thereby rendering a health problem more complex or dangerous than it otherwise would have been) because they are concerned about the testing programmes? In the light of recent developments, e.g. improved counselling and treatments which may delay the onset of AIDS, reinforcing public mistrust serves to inhibit people coming forward for care.

The guidance to nurses is quite clear (UKCC, 1993b; RCN, 1992a): when they become aware of the testing programme, they must inform patients. Thus the issue of anonymous HIV testing for seroprevalence transcends the simple gathering of data for scientific purposes. It has serious ethical and legal implications:

- Ethical implications for the role of doctors and nurses, of their duty to care and the public's trust placed in them.
- Legal implications, because there is disagreement over the position of nurses in taking samples without consent.
- Implications for the role of ethical committees, how their role and actions are made to work and how nurses contribute to them.
- Professional implications, in terms of the mode of practice – in this case authoritarian – that researchers use to relate to patients.
- Practical implications, in view of the uncertainty of the results. Is the test of value anyway in giving a real picture of the prevalence of HIV? Already, some of the less reputable sections of the popular press have suggested that HIV is a problem only for people with low moral standards living in inner-city areas. As a result, the evidence that is available runs the risk of being distorted in the face of media prejudice and irresponsibility.

How far is the research itself a symptom of the pressure within medicine to research and publish to enhance credibility and career prospects? Mihill (1991a) suggests that 'many scientists, although genuinely seeking to help, seem to regard AIDS as some exciting, state-of-the-art biomedical chess game with a particularly cunning opponent'.

It seems that the best way forward would be to divert the resources to mass public education. Nurses and doctors would have a key role to play in reaching out to people, particularly those at risk, and encouraging them to come forward for testing. Nurses especially have shown themselves to have risen to the challenge of producing excellent counselling and information-giving services. Obtaining consent from clients is part of health education, and nurses and doctors are in a unique position because of their frequent contact with the public. Simultaneously, there must be a fully resourced back-up programme of counselling and support when results are known. In this way, society gets the statistics it needs and individuals get the care they need.

HIV TESTING AND SURGERY

In the United States, one survey (New York Times, 1993) recently reported that about three-quarters of doctors and nurses were in favour of mandatory testing for surgical patients and pregnant women. More than 60% said doctors should be able to order an HIV test for patients without their consent. The majority of professionals interviewed also favoured mandatory testing for health workers.

In the UK, the debate surfaced when both the Royal College of Surgeons (RCS) and the British Orthopaedic Association (BOA) announced guidelines permitting doctors to test patients for HIV before, during or after surgery where there was a 'high degree of suspicion' that a patient was HIV positive, or where there had been a risk of transmission of blood from patient to doctor or other health workers during surgery (e.g. accidental scalpel or needlestick injury) (Mihill, 1991b).

Much of the advice looked at safety issues, and did not recommend routine testing of all patients. The chairman of the BOA said that 'we are not suggesting routine testing of every patient. That would be expensive and not very productive. But if there is any reason to believe that the patient might be HIV positive, we should have the right to test with consent. If patients refused to be tested, they would be treated as a high-risk case. We also feel that we should have the right to test with or without consent when a member of staff gets significantly contaminated with blood' (Newton, 1991). This statement summarizes the ethical minefield now being entered, and which is in many ways based on irrational thinking. For example:

- if a patient is tested and found negative, this may lead to a false sense of security. It may be that the patient is infected, but has not yet seroconverted;
- any risk of transmission of any disease can be prevented by standard universal precautions, which should be applied to all patients anyway. Raising the guard against some suspected or actual HIV-positive patients is discriminatory in the sense that it assumes other patients may be treated with few precautions. This is in the

face of evidence that patients may bear other infections, e.g. hepatitis B, which is much more easily transmitted;

- it is not clear on what basis the 'high degree of suspicion' or 'any reason to believe' which underpins the rationale for testing can be made. Inevitably this would focus once again in a discriminatory way upon perceived high-risk groups rather than those with various high-risk behaviours. Thus a patient who declares himself homosexual during the nursing assessment would be more likely to be requested to undergo a test than, say, a married man with a family in a seemingly stable relationship. This takes no account, of course, that the gay man may have been in a long-term faithful relationship, while the married man may have had multiple undisclosed and unprotected sexual experiences with others, or that his wife may have had affairs with others involving unsafe sex;
- under the concept of 'duty to care' actions taken with patients must be for their benefit. The thrust of the doctors' argument is about protecting themselves and their colleagues (even though it is based on false premises). Such actions do not therefore directly benefit the patient;
- if there are fears of transmission of HIV from patient to health worker, it would seem more appropriate to conduct a series of tests on that person rather than on the patient without consent;
- the BMA, the RCN, RCM, the National AIDS Trust and many other bodies condemned the doctors' stance as irrational, impractical and immoral. Further advice suggested that nurses must not become involved in such practices unless they are satisfied that certain conditions are being met (RCN, 1992a), for example:

  - no test should take place without the patient's consent;
  - high quality pre- and post-test counselling is available;
  - the reasons for a test being requested are clearly thought through and based on sound rationale, particularly on the need to 'identify high-risk behaviours rather than high-risk groups'.

Further support contradicting the surgeons' stance came from the legal profession, and was incorporated into UKCC guidance (UKCC, 1993b). Leaving the ethical dilemmas for nurses aside, the legality of tests of this type is extremely dubious. It was argued that 'nurses have a moral duty, and possibly even a legal duty, to intervene if surgeons attempt to carry out an HIV test for which no consent has been given' (Carlisle, 1991). Geer (1991), a lawyer with the charity Immunity, stated that 'it is proper for nurses to raise their objections and ethically they should do so'. Nurses should also avoid being 'party to the action' and being involved in taking blood samples for such tests as this was legally an assault on the patient. The UKCC (1992b) guidance is quite clear that 'On the specific issue of the taking of blood for testing without consent, the council advises all its practitioners that they expose themselves to the possibility of civil action for damages, of criminal charges of assault or of complaint to the regulatory body (the Council) alleging misconduct if they personally take the blood specimens, and of aiding and abetting an assault if they cooperate in obtaining such specimens'. The UKCC guidance describes 'exceptional circumstances' where unconsented testing may occur, but which could only be justified if they were in the interests of a particular patient at the time.

CONTACT TRACING

A major shift in the Government's testing policy took place in 1991, when the tracing of contacts of HIV-positive persons was encouraged (DoH, 1991a; Hunt, 1991), stressing that this would involve 'cooperation not coercion' and that 'confidentiality would be assured' so that people would come forward (Hunt, 1991). It was argued that, apart from epidemiological advantages, there were advantages to individual patients of knowing their HIV status. They could, for example, take steps to prevent transmission to others, improve their general health or begin monitoring and treatments which appear to delay the onset of AIDS.

Counsellors at STD clinics already discuss contact tracing with clients, but the Government statements were the first indication of a formal approval for such procedures. The advantages of contact tracing may seem to be quite obvious but, once again, this is an issue fraught with ethical, legal and practical dilemmas for nurses. Different concerns arise about tracing partners, as opposed to contact tracing of patients who, it is feared, have been infected by a health worker. The latter has been dealt with in detail above (p.51).

In January 1989 the World Health Organization (WHO) issued a consensus statement from consultation on 'partner notification' (WHO, 1989). The statement acknowledged that HIV infection differs in important ways from other sexually transmitted diseases and additional issues have to be taken into account. The purpose of partner notification is to inform people of the risks to which they have been exposed so that they can be offered counselling and other services. The WHO guidelines say that it is only acceptable if the following principles are adhered to:

• It should be in accordance with the global AIDS strategy and respect the human rights and dignity of the partners and the person who is

HIV positive. It must be part of a comprehensive programme and coordinated with other primary health-care activities, such as maternal and child health, family planning and substance abuse prevention.

- It must be voluntary and not coercive, and people must have access to services independent of their willingness to cooperate.
- The contact tracing must be confidential, concealing the identity of the person who is positive, although this has practical limitations when the person contacted has only had a single partner.
- One of the key elements in the principle stated is that it should only be undertaken when appropriate support services are available, at least counselling, the availability of testing and good-quality health and social services.

The question of resources is one immediate cause of concern. Given the long period of time during which a person may be HIV positive without any outward sign, the tracer would have to contact all sexual partners over a long period. They would also have to ask how many of them might have been intravenous drug users, or blood donors or semen donors during that period or since, and their children would have to be tested. Would they be retested, and how often, over what period?

The skills required to deal with contact tracing for a potentially fatal infection are even greater than those for other sexually transmitted diseases. A person who asks for a test at any time should be offered counselling, but what kind of counselling is given to someone who has been selected for testing on the testimony of a third party? Quite advanced skills are required.

If a patient tests HIV positive there is no problem in law for nurses in disclosing information to current or former sexual partners if the patient consents. Indeed, in most cases the nurse is reliant upon the patient for the names and addresses of contacts, and if the patient provides this information there is implied, if not expressed, consent. The problem arises when the HIV-positive patient refuses to identify names and addresses of current or former partners, and refuses to allow them to be informed. Legal advice sought by the RCN (Richmond, 1991) indicates that if nurses can be certain there is a real risk of harm to a third party (e.g. an HIV-positive person's former partner is unaware that they may be infected and may pass the virus on to others, or the patient's current partner is unaware that they may be at risk from the person) they may be able to breach patient confidentiality in order to act 'in the public interest' of another. Theoretically, the aggrieved HIV-positive person could sue the health authority for breach of confidence. In practice, it seems that the judge and/or professional conduct committee would be likely to back the nurse's decision if made in good faith and in accordance with the factors discussed above.

Contact tracing, or partner notification as it is now becoming known, is clearly fraught with difficulties, especially when the effects on the patient and partner(s) are considered of a virus that may remain asymptomatic for many years. Clearly, the effectiveness of this work is going to be underpinned by the trusting relationship which nurses can build with patients, and by their counselling and supportive skills which enable HIV-positive patients to make informed decisions. These, in the longer term, are the most effective tools to help both nurse and patient face and minimize the tremendous difficulties surrounding the issue.

LIVING WILLS

As a person progresses from being HIV positive into AIDS, the effects – physical, psychological and social – are catastrophic. The predictability, inevitability and the nature of the outcome have fuelled the debate, which has been gathering pace generally in recent years, about the degree of control people have towards the end of their life, and over the manner of ending it. Nurses are also faced with the challenge of confronting HIV = AIDS = DEATH, and helping patients to maintain control of their lives, to experience love and happiness, and to value the quality and quantity of life that remains. Nurses have therefore been drawn increasingly into the continued debate over advanced directives, or 'living wills', and euthanasia.

The BMA (British Medical Association) (1992) has decided to use the term 'advance directive' rather than living will. Their definition of the distinction is as follows:

> 'An advance directive is a mechanism whereby a competent person gives instructions about what he wishes to be done if he should subsequently lose the capacity to decide for himself. It may cover any matter upon which the individual has decided views, but is most often quoted in connection with decisions about medical treatment, particularly the treatment which might be provided as the patient approaches death. The 'living will' has a similar aim but whereas an advance directive can give instructions about any decision and can request as well as refuse specific treatments, the living will is essentially a formal declaration by a competent adult conveying his wish for any life-prolonging measures to be withheld in circumstances where there is no prospect of recovery. The object is to rebut any presumption that the patient has consented to treatment which may be administered

on the grounds of necessity. The scope of the 'living will' is therefore more limited than the advance directives and since many have shown that the term 'living will' is a misnomer and gives rise to confusion about the document's legal status in comparison with other types of will, the BMA has preferred to use the term 'advance directive'.'

An RCN document (1993b) referred to a living will as:

'...a document which attempts to set out the kind of health care that would be authorized by a patient if, at a future time, they are unable to choose, e.g. because they are unconscious, or delirious or otherwise incapacitated.

A living will is an attempt to allow patients the right to refuse treatment in advance, in case the patient is too ill to choose for themselves or becomes unable to express that choice as their condition deteriorates.'

Health-care staff, like everyone else, are subject to the law which prohibits taking steps to assist (or giving advice which would assist) another person to commit suicide. A living will cannot be a direct request to commit suicide, and if it is health-care staff must ignore that section of it.

Essentially both approaches, hereafter referred to as living wills for simplicity, seek to enable patients to control what happens to them when serious illness or death approaches. That patients should be able to direct what care they receive in such circumstances seems self-evidently to be good. However, once again an issue arises which seems at first straightforward, but is in fact loaded with ethical, practical and legal dilemmas, not least for nurses. Some organizations, to help patients, have produced guidance (Age Concern, 1988; Terrence Higgins Trust, 1992) on the format and content of a living will.

At present, however, the living will has no legal standing in the UK (although there are moves within Parliament to change this), and cannot be used to compel health workers to act in a particular way. Both the RCN and the BMA have initially rejected legalization of living wills, preferring instead to maintain a degree of clinical freedom to allow health-care workers to take account of the patient's wishes but not automatically follow them, in the light of changing circumstances at the time.

The living will can only convey the state of mind of the patient at the time and may be based on patients' perceptions of their own self-worth and self-esteem – requesting no active treatment, for example, because of long-term influences that have led them to feel unworthy or without value as a person. There are also problems in ensuring that the will is unambiguous, that it has not been produced under the undue influence of others, or that it is outdated, the patient having had a change of mind but not changed the document.

Although the absence of legal support for the living will provide scope for professional judgement, a nurse may find difficulties arising if the will is not accepted. Such a refusal may damage the trust that the patient has in the nurse. On the other hand, legalizing such documents may indicate that 'allowing people to die, rather than continuing to look after them, is the cheaper option and there will be grave suspicion of any government that supports this kind of act. The argument could also influence the patient himself, who sees his family's resources being eaten up by his terminal care and feels obliged to ask for termination' (Andrews, 1990).

Ethical dilemmas about treatment at the end of life are made worse by poor communications: doctors not making their decisions clear to nurses, or nurses not discussing reasons for requests with patients or relatives. It is here that Wells' (1988) assertion that nurses must first of all be able to sort out their own moral codes and value systems if they are to be able to help others, is seen to be valid. The nurse who has prejudicial feelings about people who have HIV/AIDS is not going to be able to act in the patient's best interests and give advocacy and support effectively.

It is perhaps as well to remember that no document is a substitute for a good nurse–patient relationship based on trust.

EUTHANASIA

Under English law a person who aids, abets, counsels or procures the suicide of another, or an attempt by another to commit suicide, shall be liable to conviction or indictment to imprisonment for a term not exceeding 14 years (Suicide Act 1961). A full discussion of euthanasia is beyond the scope of this text, but a number of issues will be raised here, not least because euthanasia is sometimes seen as an option when 'one can still, in this day and age, die in agony and that a tortured, hopeless life is cruel and utterly pointless' (Bogarde, 1991). Kennedy, a prominent advocate of euthanasia, argues that the law should be changed to allow a 'qualified member of the medical profession to assist a patient to die' (Kennedy, 1990).

The illnesses that strike with AIDS can indeed be most 'tortured' and 'cruel', and nurses are often the frontline workers supporting patients and families in their distress. In The Netherlands, steps have already been taken to legalize medical participation in euthanasia under certain circumstances, but this has led to the worst fears of some being realized, as the number of cases of 'mercy killings' subsequently escalated.

Requests for euthanasia may often be based on misconceptions about terminal care, the nature of pain relief and other support available, as well as an individual's perceptions of self-worth. Life which is 'utterly pointless' to one person may be valuable to another, however many limitations or however much suffering is involved. Furthermore, perceptions about dying may change over time. A healthy young person may express a preference for euthanasia at the thought of illness which leads to dependence on others. However, when the circumstances actually arise the view may change, with life being seen as worth clinging to whatever its quality or quantity.

In contrast to the proponents of euthanasia, others have argued that nurses should have no part in it (RCN, 1992b), not only because of the legal implications for themselves but also because they would undermine the essential trust in the nurse–patient relationship: workers normally associated with healing would become associated with killing. Pollard (1991) believes euthanasia to be equivalent to homicide or infanticide. He fears a 'slippery slope' phenomenon, where eugenics based on different sociological as well as economic criteria will then become acceptable. Patients such as those with HIV and AIDS would be more at risk of being 'encouraged' to die because of the stigmatization they already endure. Euthanasia would be a redundant concept if improvements were continued in the control of pain and the promotion of dignity in palliative care: 'At the end of life, patients need comfort, and not torments such as the fear of being killed' (Pollard, 1991).

Further distinctions have been drawn between active (i.e. injecting a lethal drug) and passive euthanasia: withholding a treatment so that 'nature takes its course'. Although it could be argued that while the actions in either case are different, the intent remains the same, i.e. to kill. Furthermore, a distinction has also been made between giving a treatment with the intention of relieving suffering (e.g. a morphine injection) which may have the secondary effect of shortening life, and giving a lethal injection with the first intention of ending life. These issues were brought to the fore in 1992 in two much-publicized cases, one related to a doctor, Nigel Cox, who gave a lethal injection to a terminally ill patient, and the other to a patient, Anthony Bland, who had been in a persistent vegetative state for 3 years. In the Cox case (1992) the doctor was convicted of attempted murder but received a 1-year suspended sentence, was reprimanded by the General Medical Council (although his name remained on the register) and returned to his employment under a period of suspension. This relatively light sentence conveyed a considerable degree of sympathy for the doctor's position. Interestingly, it was the nurse who (quite correctly, according to her Code of Conduct) reported the doctor's actions who was vilified in the press as treacherous and uncaring.

In the Bland case, the court ruled that artificial feeding was a medical treatment and could be discontinued; the patient subsequently died (Airedale v. Bland, 1993). The court case appeared to have taken little account of the nursing perspective or the support nurses needed once the feeding of Mr Bland was ordered to be discontinued (Wright, 1993).

The debate over the rights and wrongs of euthanasia continues, but from this discussion it seems that certain legal requirements constrain nurses. Those who choose to act outside these constraints must reflect carefully upon their values and actions and be prepared for the consequences of their acts outside the law. Meeting the patient's wishes, ensuring that these are based on informed decision making, keeping legal requirements in mind and making their own moral and practical judgements is a difficult balancing act which euthanasia brings into sharp focus. The nurse's duty to act in the patient's best interest may be difficult when there are different perceptions of what their best interests are, and when the law lays down a set of rules which may conflict with the nurse's and patient's ethical stances.

CONCLUSION

That which is legal is not necessarily ethical, and vice versa. As is illustrated by the above discussion, nurses are at the forefront of this conflict. For example:

- a nurse may support a patient's wish for the means to end life, and in conscience accepts this as the most ethical approach in this particular patient's best interest. But the law forbids acts of euthanasia;
- a patient may find cannabis the best recourse for relief of pain and anxiety in terminal illness. The nurse may agree that this is in the best interest of the patient, but to procure it or encourage its use is outside the law;
- the law may permit certain forms of testing or the breaching of confidence, but the nurse may find such actions incompatible with his or her ethical framework.

Many such examples can be identified in the work involved in caring for people who are HIV positive or who have AIDS. Sometimes the issues are made more confusing by media hypocrisy, the prejudice of colleagues or Government indecision. For example, the *Health of the Nation* policy (DoH, 1993b) exhorts nurses to help reduce the incidence of HIV and teenage pregnancy, yet there are legal constraints on what they can tell children about homosexual lifestyles, and local education policies may restrict their access to children and what can be taught.

An enormous amount depends upon nurses, how they act out their own values and perceive their own roles. Codes of practice and professional recommendations offer standards of good practice with HIV and AIDS patients, and proscribe those who act judgementally or in a discriminatory fashion. It is difficult, however, for nurses to conceal their own values and act always in the patient's best interest. Hypocrisy has a way of revealing itself, and so nurses who transmit their moralizing on to the lives of their patients may not only fail in 'beneficence' but may actually do harm. For example, there is abundant evidence to show that patients who do not have a therapeutic relationship with their nurse are more likely to be demoralized and deteriorate and die earlier. Beneficence and non-maleficence, the duty to do good and to prevent harm, underpin the nurse–patient relationship. It is in the nurse–patient relationship where these values can be acted out and which forms the battleground between ethics and the law, between personal morals and public duty.

It is quite clear what patients expect from nurses. They expect them to be on their side, to be among those who act on their behalf when they are unable to do so themselves, to offer compassion and consideration amid the most profound of illness experiences. Nurses are needed as a 'presence' with patients, bearing witness to their health problems and helping them through them (Benner, 1984). As companions in health care (Campbell, 1984) they can build a relationship based on trust, respect and competence, which is itself healing. Nurses can then not only help patients to 'get better', they can also help them 'feel better' (Kitson, 1988), and the latter may be the most important when death is inevitable. Nurses fail in these when they permit conscience to be blurred by prejudice or beneficence to be clouded by moralizing and discrimination.

The best interest of patients lie, in part, with empowered nurses who are clear and assertive about their roles and responsibilities, reflective on the practice and in tune with their own consciences. Such nurses are best placed, as Boyd (1993) suggests, to find their way with their patients through the ethical dilemmas that face them.

REFERENCES

Age Concern (1988) *The Living Will: Consent to Treatment at the End of Life*, Arnold, London.

Airedale NHS Trust (Respondents) v. Bland (Acting by his guardian ad litem) (Appelant) (1993). House of Lords, London 4.2.93.

Akinsanya, J. and Rouse, P. (1992) Who will care? a survey of knowledge and attitudes of hospital nurses to people with HIV and AIDS. *Journal of Advanced Nursing*, **17**, 400–1.

Andrews, J. (1990) The ultimate choice. *Nursing Times*, **86**(12), 18.

Atkinson, J. (1991) cited in Hand, D. (1991) To test or not to test. *Nursing Standard*, **5**(46), 17–19.

Benner, P. (1984) *From Novice to Expert*, Addison Wesley, New York.

Bogarde, D. (1991) cited in Ellis, P. (1991) Living wills to end life. *Nursing Standard*, **5**(26), 18–19.

Boyd, K. (1993) Euthanasia: back to the future. *Bulletin of Medical Ethics*, **88**, 25–32.

British Medical Association (1992) *BMA Statement on Advanced Directives*, BMA, London.

British Medical Journal (1991) Prison for refusing to tell. *British Medical Journal*, **303**, 206.

Bulletin of Medical Ethics (1992) D. Cox. *BME*, November, **83**, 4.

Campbell, A. V. (1984) *Moderated Love*, SPCK, London.

Carlisle, D. (1991) Lawyer specifies moral duty in HIV testing. *Nursing Times*, **87**(11), 7.

Connor, S. (1994) Papering over the pain. *The Independent*, 2.1.94, 12–13.

Department of Health (1988) *Goverment Announces New Steps to Monitor the Spread of HIV Infection*, DoH, London.

Department of Health (1991a) *Contact Tracing – Press Statement*, Department of Health, January 1991.

Department of Health (1991b) *AIDS–HIV Infected Health Care Workers*, HMSO, London.

Department of Health (1993a) *HIV-Infected Health Care Workers* – Press release. DoH, London.

Department of Health (1993b) *Health of the Nation: The Contribution of Nurses, Midwives and Health Visitors*, HMSO, London.

Department of Health and Welsh Office (1987) *Short Term Prediction of HIV Infection and AIDS in England and Wales*. Report of a Working Group. HMSO, London.

de Selincourt, K. A. (1992) A breach of trust? *Nursing Times*, **88**, 11–19.

Emson, H. E. (1989) Secret HIV testing of babies. *Institute of Medical Ethics Bulletin*.

Frank, A. (1991) *At the Will of the Body*, Houghton Mifflin, Boston.

Geer, D. (1991) cited in Carlisle, D. (1991) Lawyer specifies moral duty in HIV testing. *Nursing Times*, **87**(11), 7.

Hand, D. (1991) To test or not to test. *Nursing Standard*, **5**(46), 17–19.

Hansard (1993) Parliamentary report 26.4.93, Cols. 280-1. HMSO, London.

Hunt, L. (1991) HIV victims to be questioned over partners. *The Independent*, 1.12.91, p.3.

Illman, J. (1993) History lesson. *Nursing Times*, **89**(26), 26–8.

Ingrams, R. (1990) *The Observer*, 12.9.90, 12.

Institute of Medical Ethics (1988) Babies tested secretly for AIDS. *Institute of Medical Ethics Bulletin*, 3.6.89.

Kennedy, L. (1990) *Euthanasia – the Good Death*, Chatto and Windus, London.

Keyser, D. (1989) Selecting a strategy: some questions to be asked and answered, in *Changing nursing practice*, (ed S.G. Wright), Arnold, London, pp.12–14.

Kitson, A. (1988) On the concept of nursing care, in *Ethical Issues in Caring*, (eds G. Fairbairn and S. Fairbairn), Gower, Aldershot.

Mackereth, P. (1993) *'Otherness' – a Critical Analysis of Autonomy in Relationship to AIDS, Advocacy and Homophobia*. Unpublished MA thesis, University of Keele.

Medical Research Council (1988) *A Programme of Epidemiological Research Based on Named and Anonymous HIV Testing for HIV Infection*. Report to the Department of Health (S/819/230), HMSO, London.

Menzies, I. (1961) The functioning of social systems as a defence against anxiety, in *Containing Anxiety in Institutions*, (ed I. Menzies-Lyth), Free Association Books, London.

Mihill, C. A. (1991a) A deadly decision. *The Guardian*, 26.6.91.

Mihill, C. A. (1991b) Patients face AIDS test before surgery. *The Guardian*, 7.1.91.

National Federation for Education Research (1993) *Nursing and AIDS: material matters*, NFER Nelson, Slough.

Newton, G. (1991) cited in Mihill, C. A. (1991b) Patients face AIDS test before surgery. *The Guardian*, 7.1.91.

New York Times (1993) Survey finds doctors and nurses in favour of taking tests for AIDS. *New York Times*, 15.6.93.

Patton, C. (1990) *Inventing AIDS*, Routledge, London.

Pollard, B. (1991) *Euthanasia: Should We Kill the Dying?* Little Hills Press, Bedford.

Pratt, R. (1986) *AIDS: a Strategy for Nursing Care*, Arnold, London.

Richmond, H. (1991) *Contact Tracing re HIV/AIDS*, Report to the Royal College of Nursing Ethics Committee, RCN, London.

Royal College of Nursing (1985) Press release. RCN, London, 10 January 1985.

Royal College of Nursing (1991) *Contact Tracing re HIV/AIDS*, RCN, London.

Royal College of Nursing (1992a) *RCN Briefing on HIV and Antibody Tests*, RCN, London.

Royal College of Nursing (1992b) *Position Statement on Euthanasia*, RCN, London.

Royal College of Nursing (1993a) *Refusal to nurse: guidance for nurses*. Issues in Nursing and Health No. 18. RCN, London.

Royal College of Nursing (1993b) *Living Wills: Guidance for Nurses*. Issues in Nursing and Health No. 14, revised 1993. RCN, London.

Royal College of Nursing (1992) *Report on UKCC Revised Guidance and HIV infection*, RCN, London.

Salvage, J. (1986) *The Politics of Nursing*, Heinemann, London.

Terrence Higgins Trust (1992) *What's a Living Will?* Terrence Higgins Trust, London.

United Kingdom Central Council for Nursing, Midwifery and Health Visiting (1991) Transcript of the Professional Conduct Committee. UKCC, London.

United Kingdom Central Council for Nursing, Midwifery and Health Visiting (1992a) *Code of Professional Conduct*, UKCC, London.

United Kingdom Central Council for Nursing, Midwifery and Health Visiting (1992b) *Council's Position on Acquired Immune Deficiency Syndrome and Human Immuno-deficiency Virus Infection*, UKCC, London. Registrar's letter No. 8/1992.

United Kingdom Central Council for Nursing, Midwifery and Health Visiting (1993a) *Consultation on the Council's Proposed Standards for Post-Registration Education*, UKCC, London. Registrar's letter No. 8/1993.

United Kingdom Central Council for Nursing, Midwifery and Health Visiting. (1993b) *Anonymous Testing for the Prevalence of the Human Immuno-deficiency Virus*, UKCC, London. Registrar's letter No. 12/1993.

United Kingdom Central Council for Nursing, Midwifery and Health Visiting (1993c) *Acquired Immune Deficiency Syndrome and Human Immuno-deficiency Virus Infection*, UKCC, London. Registrar's letter No. 12/93.

Wells, R. (1988) Ethics and information. *Senior Nurse*, **8**(6), 8–10.

World Health Organization (1989) *Global Programme on AIDS and Programmes of STD: Consensus Statement from Consultation on Partner Notification for Preventing HIV Transmission*, WHO, Geneva.

Wright, S. G. (1993) What makes a person? *Nursing Times*, **89**(21), 42–5.

The education debate   5

Carol Pellowe

INTRODUCTION

In the early years of the epidemic, the nursing profession was neither equipped nor prepared to cope. AIDS had been seen as an American problem which would remain there, and no attempts had been made within Colleges of Nursing to address it. The main source of information was the media, whose attention focused on the highly infectious nature of this disease and, as Wells (1987) notes: 'Nurses are consumers of the media, too, and have interpreted such information in their provision of care'. Consequently, this highly vulnerable group of people suffered at the hands of those from whom they expected care and support and, once again, nurse educators have fought a rearguard action to limit the damage.

The challenge of nurse education is to ensure that all nurses are thoroughly cognizant of the issues so that they can deliver competent and compassionate care. As we enter the second decade of this epidemic, it is useful to take stock of progress to date.

NURSES' ATTITUDES TO HIV

'Each registered nurse, midwife and health visitor is accountable for his or her practice and, in the exercise of professional accountability shall: act always in such a way as to promote and safeguard the wellbeing and interest of patients/clients and ensure that no action or omission on their part, within their sphere of influence, is detrimental to the condition or safety of their patients/clients' (UKCC, 1992).

Nurses are the frontline caregivers, and consequently can have a significant impact on the length and quality of a patient's life. Yet, despite the UKCC's Code of Professional Conduct, through either ignorance, fear or prejudice, good care has not always been proffered. Consideration of the research on nurses' attitudes helps to identify areas of concern.

Blumenfield *et al.* (1987) found that two-thirds of nurses reported that their families and friends had reacted to their caring for HIV-infected individuals by treating them as if they themselves were infected; 50% expressed fear of caring for male homosexuals, believing that HIV infection could occur through casual contact, despite universal infection control precautions, faith in which seems to be uncertain. Wiley and Acklin (1988) found that nurses preferred all patients to be serologically tested on admission (75%) and the results of antibody testing to be made available to all personnel involved in care (87%). With this information, 54% believed that all nurses should be entitled to refuse to care for patients with HIV-related illnesses.

Bond *et al.* (1990a, b) published two papers on community staff in England and Wales and, later, in Scotland. At present, HIV experience in the community is limited and this was found to be a major cause for concern. Staff need to be assisted to make links between the knowledge they possess and its application to caring for those with HIV disease, and in developing and practising skills. A simple 10-question multiple-choice questionnaire revealed a glaring void in knowledge. In the English survey, only three questions were answered correctly by more than 75% of respondents. Both surveys showed a clear gradient in refusals to care against people's lifestyle: 'The association between a belief in the right to refuse to care and concern about the lack of knowledge indicates the powerful role that fear may be playing in influencing personal beliefs about certain patient groups and about dealing with infected patients'.

Another key issue was confidentiality and the right to know people's HIV status: 78% of respondents in the survey in Scotland felt that they should be informed of a patient's status without that patient's consent. This 'undermines the possibility for positive relationships with patients. If those who are at risk of infection or who are infected cannot be sure of confidentiality about their HIV status, this will surely discourage them from coming forward for testing and to seek care'.

Within hospitals the situation is depressingly similar, as Akinsanya and Rouse (1991) identified. Not only did this show a deficit of knowledge – for example, 24% of respondents agreed that there was a degree of risk of infection through insect bites, but also 37% were in favour of the right to refuse to care. In summary, the report noted that 'nurses working in hospitals are not sufficiently knowledgeable about the infection nor well prepared to meet the challenge of caring for people with AIDS', and this was as we entered the second decade of the epidemic.

However, the fault does not lie entirely with the care providers, as shown by Faltermeyer (1990). In his survey, he found that few nurses had tried to improve their knowledge, but this equally applied to nurse teachers, the very people who are expected to give accurate and current knowledge to others. The level of knowledge between learners and qualified nurses did not appear to be significantly different, and this is particularly disturbing as the profession moves into the era of self-directed study and individuals taking responsibility for their own professional development.

'As nurses move rapidly into the field of health promotion and education, the urgent need to improve their educational knowledge must be met with a commitment from managerial staff to improve motivation and knowledge by ensuring that qualified staff are positively encouraged to update their knowledge.'

The need for education about HIV and AIDS is clear; however, it must not be addressed in isolation but as a part of holistic care.

THE ISSUES

In constructing educational initiatives on HIV and AIDS, it is important to be clear about one's aims. There is nothing fundamentally different about caring for someone with HIV disease as the nursing care is the same as for any other patient. It is the issues surrounding the patient's condition that create the difficulties that need to be addressed. These include sensitive areas which have traditionally been ignored in nurse education, such as sexuality, loss and drug use, while claiming to offer holistic care. McHaffie (1993) noted: 'There is little evidence that the matter of patients' sexuality has been addressed adequately – whether it is applied to heterosexuals or homosexuals. And death and dying remain problem areas for many practitioners. Even those who were frequently exposed to people dying at relatively young ages spoke eloquently of their own difficulties in dealing with dying at such close quarters.'

The ENB Course No. 934 (now Post Registration Award) 'The Care and Management of People with AIDS and HIV', succinctly itemizes the key issues as follows:

- the disease;
- associated research and other relevant information;
- assessing the psychosocial, physical and pastoral needs of the patient/client, family groups and others;
- planning, implementing and evaluating appropriate care programmes;

- developing self-awareness in relation to sexuality and personal attitudes and prejudices;
- counselling and supporting the patient, partner, family groups and others, including colleagues;
- the process of grief;
- utilizing available relevant statutory voluntary agencies;
- preventing and controlling infection, including surveillance and control action;
- promoting health education;
- maintaining confidentiality;
- ethical considerations and conflicts.

This outline curriculum was published in 1988, and one could be forgiven for wondering what progress, if any, has been made in the interim. Yet the above still constitute the key focus of any HIV education initiative. The main problem remains the low number of nurses receiving this input and subsequently being supported in incorporating their skills and knowledge into their practice. Although there has been a significant increase in the variety and number of ENB 934 courses available across the country, only a tiny proportion of the total nursing population will ever have access to one; it is therefore nonsensical to rely on these courses as a solution to all problems. Every institution involved in nurse education or health-care provision must become 'HIV aware' and develop a comprehensive educational strategy which influences preregistration courses, post-basic courses and staff development opportunities.

In many areas, Project 2000 is fully implemented and should adequately cover the issues, although concrete evidence of its effects is awaited. The first results are to be found in the evaluation by the National Foundation for Educational Research of the educational material on HIV available to teachers and their decision-making processes in its selection (1993). This highlighted poor adherence to the adoption of universal infection control precautions, with subsequent breaches in patient confidentiality, and recommended that nurse educators at preregistration level review the attention paid to these areas throughout the course. In colleges awaiting Project 2000 validation and funding, curricular development has taken place to introduce an HIV thread, or to upgrade their current course to diploma level, in which case a more radical approach has been possible. In the early 1980s, the first educational response to HIV was its inclusion as a disease process, ignoring the underlying issues such as communication skills, sexuality or stigma. This is not surprising, as traditional formats of nurse education have never adequately addressed these areas. As Savage (1987) notes, it was assumed that nurses' experience as students would be sufficient to enable them to come to terms with their own emotions, uncertainties and identities. Now, a more psychosocial approach is adopted, which allows for the development of communication skills, the consideration of ethics and philosophy, and the exploration of sexuality.

All these exciting and important changes in preregistration will come to nothing unless there is a commitment to ongoing staff development, for the majority of nurses are already qualified. The Riverside Health Authority and College of Health Studies made a commitment in 1988 to provide HIV education and training for all staff. Consequently, all new staff underwent an HIV awareness day as part of their orientation programme. All post-registration clinical courses included HIV and its impact upon that specialty, and tailor-made courses were provided for specific service areas, e.g. substance misuse, midwifery and community nursing. For those who had completed the ENB Course no.934, there was the opportunity every year to attend an update day, which highlighted significant changes in treatment and care provision. The strategy was to highlight the significance of HIV to the service wherever possible, and bring to the attention of nursing staff the HIV Ethical Framework (Riverside Health Authority, 1990), which explained the policy statements relating to HIV disease. Without this strategy, it would not have been possible to provide competent, cognizant and confident care.

THE PRESENT AND THE FUTURE

Many changes are currently taking place in nurse education, bringing about a great deal of uncertainty; it is therefore remarkable that HIV education should continue to develop, yet significant developments are taking place that deserve attention.

THE NEED FOR A CAREER PATHWAY IN HIV NURSING

With the creation of dedicated HIV units, it was evident that nurses would elect to work in this area long term. There is now a need to retain and professionally develop these nurses. The Framework is one option which is practice-based, but there are others.

ENB FRAMEWORK FOR CONTINUING PROFESSIONAL EDUCATION AND THE HIGHER AWARD

In 1989, over 238 000 nurses, midwives and health visitors were practising in the NHS in England and Wales, of whom only one in five possessed a post-registration certificate for the area in which they practised. The provision of post-basic education was sketchy, uncoordinated and unhelpfully split between what was recordable and what was in-service training. Both were considered to contribute to professional development, and should be recognized in one system. In order to address these problems and make the best use of resources, in the spring of 1992 the ENB introduced the Framework, leading to the ENB Higher Award. Its focus is the development of the individual in conjunction with service managers and the providers of education. It is open to all practitioners whose names appear on the Professional Register, and is particularly attractive to those who are clinically based. The Framework allows practitioners to develop clinical career pathways, and for those who wish to achieve the Higher Award there are the 10 Key Characteristics to be mastered and incorporated into practice.

In the first wave of institutions approved to implement the Framework consideration was given to their higher education link, as the Higher Award is an integrated award of professional and academic study which carries the status of at least a first honours degree. The system also demanded that the institution be able to manage credit accumulation and transfer (CATS), which in turn required the ability to assess prior learning, whether it be formal or experiential.

Colleges already offering Project 2000 courses, and therefore established with a higher institution, were in the best position to develop the Framework. Those offering the ENB Course no.934 found this an opportunity to develop the ENB Course no.280, 'The Care and Provision for People with HIV and AIDS'. This is a modularized course where members choose two modules from the choice of clinical, management or education. On completion of this and possession of the ENB 934, they can register a qualification in AIDS patient care. The irony is that theoretically, by opting for the latter two modules (management and education), one could achieve this without ever having nursed a patient with HIV disease. Other options currently being pursued include the development of HIV modules within a diploma framework. The University of the South Bank offers a Diploma in Higher Education (Health Studies) as part of its INSET framework. This has proved attractive to Colleges of Health Studies as it is flexible and incorporates a wide variety of modules, so that health-care workers can choose a tailor-made pathway. This might include clinical ENB-validated courses as well as those with a professional development focus. At Thames Valley University, two courses focus on developing clinical practice in caring for those with HIV disease. The first is the ENB 934, which includes an assessment in line with the ENB circular 1992/28/RLV, and carries two credits at level 2. The second is 'Developing practice in the care and management of people with HIV disease', which is worth three credits at level 2. The purpose of this course is to explore the issues associated with HIV disease at a greater depth and apply this knowledge to practice. Within this course there is the opportunity for students to spend time on a project placement, the purpose of which is to consolidate their knowledge in their chosen topic area. During the first module, students negotiate a learning contract which specifies the intended learning outcomes of the placement.

In order to complete this diploma, students can credit prior learning and/or choose from a range of non-clinical modules, which include management, health education, communication skills, and teaching and assessing. The opportunity to study with a multiprofessional group representing a diversity of experience is highly attractive to students, and enhances the learning milieu.

A third option is to elect for a sexual health pathway. In response to the Government's document *Health of the Nation; First Steps for the NHS* (DoH, 1992), which targeted the promotion of sexual health, some colleges have developed a specific sexual health course which includes HIV and the ENB course no.276, parts one and two. The course currently being offered by Princess Alexandra and Newham College of Nursing and Midwifery is an example of this and can be studied to degree level.

From these options it is evident that significant developments have taken place in the field of HIV education. None of the above are mutually exclusive, and within the next 3 years the scope of courses, as well as their availability, should increase. The unknown factor is the extent to which services will support education and sanction study leave. The salad days of extensive study leave are over. Staff applying for leave need to be clear about the relevance of their proposal to their work situation and be prepared to contribute to it either financially or during time off. The modularization of courses has enabled students to elect their own pace of study and, where appropriate, to take a break. What remains abundantly clear is that continuing education is here to stay, and all nurses need to take note and get involved.

Sexual health and the reflective practitioner constitute the buzzwords of the 1990s, yet unless they are taken seriously and developed, a major learning opportunity will have been lost. It is essential to understand these concepts and incorporate them into courses.

The *Health of the Nation* Green Paper, published in June 1991, identified the need to concentrate on health promotion and, in the national targets published the following year, sexual health was mentioned in terms of the need to reduce the incidence of gonorrhoea and the number of teenage pregnancies. Within the strategy, recommendations are made for each level of service, e.g. RHA corporate contracts should 'review the provision of, and if appropriate agree a strategy for, the development of education and training for all professionals involved in promoting sexual health' and provide unit business plans to 'establish continuing staff training programmes in HIV/AIDS and sexual health'.

However, the promotion of sexual health in a positive light requires an understanding of sexuality, an area which has largely been ignored. The Department of Health and the ENB agreed to co-host two workshops in order to 'prepare a report on the basis of a consultative process on what the problems and challenges are of raising awareness of sexuality into multiprofessional training'. The objectives for the workshops were:

- to establish why an understanding of sexuality is required in health and social care;
- to examine the problems inherent in providing sexuality education and training for health-care professionals, and to identify practice examples;
- to identify strategies to effect an increased knowledge base and change of attitude towards sexuality education and training as it relates to health-care practice.

Each workshop was attended by 40 invited participants, who were subsequently subdivided into four groups to tackle the issues of Why, Who, How and What. Valuable preparatory work was achieved during these workshops, the results of which were reported at a conference in London in March 1993. Since then, the ENB commissioned and have published an open learning pack: *Caring for people with sexually transmitted diseases, including HIV disease*, and guidelines: *Sexual health education and training: guidelines for good practice in the teaching of nurses, midwives and health visitors*. A follow-up conference organized by the ENB was held in Cambridge in June 1994, where both publications were introduced. The need to include sexuality and sexual health into current curricula, and the development of supportive training for teachers in this area, were highlighted as high priorities if the Government's targets are to be realized.

Reflection and reflective practice came to the attention of nurse educationalists in the mid-1980s with the publication of the Project 2000 documents (UKCC, 1985). Despite the attention it has received, few nurses proudly declare themselves to be 'reflective practitioners', largely because there is confusion as to what it entails. Newell (1992) maintains that this is largely due to the lack of critical examination of either the theoretical or the practical problems of reflection and the vagueness surrounding how to do it. Boud *et al.* (1985) view it as deliberate learning which is focused primarily on experience. Following an experience the student reconsiders the events that contributed to that experience, and it is this reprocessing that contributes to learning. Throughout an average day most people will reflect on incidents, often unconsciously, but 'Reflection in the context of learning is a generic term for those intellectual and affective activities in which individuals engage to explore their experiences in order to lead to new understandings and appreciations. It can be done well or badly, successfully or unsuccessfully'. The important thing is to concentrate on how best those involved can benefit.

Jarvis (1992) believes that 'professional practice is about meaningful conscious action in a specific field and seeking to learn from practice and so improve it constantly, and so become experts'. Herein lies a potential pitfall, as the experts may become 'habitualized' in their practice and resistant to change, in which case ritual takes precedence. The influence of learners in a practice environment is often a stimulus to staff, particularly for those who act as preceptors, but Jarvis notes two essential ingredients: first, the need to help practitioners to read more purposefully and manage their own learning, which he believes is the manager's responsibility; and secondly, there must be time to reflect so that the learning opportunity is not lost. If time is not available, he warns, 'it will be an occupation determined exclusively by business concerns'. This would appear to be a particularly timely reminder. In summary, Jarvis sees two elements to encouraging reflective practice in the profession. Nursing needs its own theory of practice and everyone needs training in how to reflect on their own practice and to support others in theirs.

POST-REGISTRATION EDUCATION AND PRACTICE (PREP)

The final piece in the educational jigsaw is PREP. Following on from the work undertaken for Project 2000, the UKCC set up the Post-Registration Education and Practice Project, or PREPP, which reported in 1990. In order to make post-registration education relevant, responsive and cost-effective, it proposed a three-tier approach. The first level would be primary practice, which follows on immediately from initial registration and incorporates a period of supervised practice by a preceptor. One then has the opportunity to undertake further study to become a specialist, and ultimately an advanced practitioner. The UKCC has just published its consultation document on proposed standards for post-registration education (UKCC, 1993). It proposes that a programme leading to specialist (or, in the case of midwives, enhanced) practitioner should be no less than the equivalent of 6 months' full-time study at the academic level of at least a first degree. To become an advanced practitioner, it suggests a further 3 months' full-time equivalent study, also at level 3. Considering that these courses could not be taken consecutively, as practitioners would need time to adjust to their specialist role before pursuing further studies, it is disappointing that the advanced course is not at least at Master's level.

For those already with a specialist qualification there will be automatic crediting arrangements in the first 5 years, except for enrolled nurses whose specialist course did not enable them to attain a first-level qualification. During the same period there will be the chance to credit unlimited previous learning towards a specialist qualification. If this proposal is accepted, those in possession of a good professional portfolio can look forward to a new status overnight. For those in less enviable positions the outlook is not so rosy. Enrolled nurses will continue to struggle to find a conversion course, and those not wishing to convert must content themselves with primary practice. Nurses who registered before Project 2000 will need to adapt to degree-level courses without the experience of a diploma-level study. This, of course, assumes that their manager approves the study application, for in this new age of contracting, education will be purchaser led.

Increasingly, purchasers will be individual nurses taking responsibility for their own professional development. With the above constraints, the use of open and distance learning will become ever more popular. The ENB pack is a beginning and moves are already afoot by universities to incorporate it into Higher Award frameworks. What has yet to be identified is the amount of tutorial support and encouragement really needed by someone using this pack.

In the arena of HIV education there will be considerable activity, for not only will all ENB Post-Registration Award no.934 courses have to be upgraded to level 3, but possession of the no.934 and two modules of the ENB 280 will not of itself constitute a specialist practitioner's qualification. Forty days represents the current minimum time to achieve this, which is considerably short of the 6 months that the UKCC recommends. None of this should daunt educationalists, but clear thinking about purchasers' requirements should be to the fore when contemplating change.

The standards set for teachers of nursing and midwifery are probably of much more concern. The UKCC is proposing that teachers should not only be graduates and hold a teaching qualification, but that they 'must possess and maintain relevant and up-to-date clinical experience; relevant and up-to-date subject experience; a higher level of knowledge than the student; and the ability to teach effectively through a variety of methods'! As Colleges of Nursing and Health Studies negotiate their entry into institutions of higher education, they would be well advised to take note of this.

No matter how exciting and important these proposals may seem, one should not overlook the suggestion in the document that the vast majority of nurses will remain in primary practice. This may be through choice or for lack of alternatives. Either way, their gateway to developing professional knowledge and clinical competence is the mandatory five study days over a 3-year period. If these are to be the frontline deliverers of care, the need to examine and plan carefully the content of these days is critical. Regrettably, it seems that the UKCC does not wish to have these validated for fear of restricting choice.

THE WAY AHEAD

Nursing education, like the rest of the NHS, is undergoing a period of turmoil and change. Yet never before has the need to be focused and clear about one's aims been so crucial. The HIV pandemic will be with us to the end of this century and beyond, and though the numbers infected and requiring care in the UK may be fewer than originally anticipated, the need for education does not lessen. Over the next 5 years there will be a shift in client groups from gay men to, in effect, the rest of the population. This will create dilemmas for nurses, especially for those in preregistration, as many come into the profession because they want to care for and help the sick, yet people with HIV-related illnesses present them with a different challenge. These people have an illness which is also a social issue. Some are seen as 'innocent', whereas others 'have brought it upon themselves'. As the epidemic affects more heterosexual men and women, who will help the nurses to reconcile their fears and prejudices and empower them in their personal lives?

The hope is that the caring profession of nursing will value its members enough to provide them with help and protection at every opportunity. To date, the evidence for this has been patchy. If HIV education is going to be addressed, three issues appear paramount:

1. There must be a joint responsibility for professional development between education and service management. PREP may create the necessary partnership, but unless joint responsibility is adopted training will remain ad hoc and inadequate.

2. HIV education needs to be brought into line with mainstream nurse education and constitute one aspect of a programme in sexual health. This would give maximum exposure to the topic, avoid repetition and enable students to appreciate sexual health in its broadest scope. In order to achieve this, considerable preparation of teaching staff will be required but this would be in line with the UKCC recommended standards.

3. Staff support must become something of real meaning and value. As we encourage staff to reflect upon their practice and develop, we cannot shirk the responsibility of allowing them a safe place to share their dilemmas.

As the epidemic changes, so must educational initiatives. It could be that in 5 years' time we will face a different set of issues, but this should not deter course planners as we know that progress in some areas has kept pace and will continue to do so.

REFERENCES

Akinsanya, J.A. and Rouse, P.I. (1991) *Who Will Care? A Survey of the Knowledge and Attitudes of Hospital Nurses to People with HIV/AIDS*, Faculty of Health and Social Work, Anglia Polytechnic.

Blumenfield, M., Smith, P.J. and Milazzo, J. (1987) Survey of attitudes of nurses working with AIDS patients. *General Hospital Psychiatry*, **9**, 58–63.

Bond, S., Rhodes, T. and Setters, J. (1990a) HIV infection and AIDS in England: the experience, knowledge and intentions of community nursing staff. *Journal of Advanced Nursing*, **15**, 249–55.

Bond, S., Rhodes, T. and Philips, P. (1990b) Knowledge and attitudes. *Nursing Times*, **86**(45), 49–51.

Boud, D., Keogh, R. and Walker, D. (1985) *Reflection: Turning Experience into Learning*, Kogan Page, London.

Department of Health (1992) *Health of the Nation; First Steps for the NHS*, HMSO, London.

Department of Health (1993) *Education for Sexual Health and Sexuality: a Report of Workshops*, HMSO, London.

English National Board (1991) *Framework for Continuing Professional Education for Nurses, Midwives and Health Visitors, Guide to Implementation*.

Faltermeyer, T.S. (1990) Nursing knowledge about AIDS in the UK. *AIDS Patient Care*, **4**(6), 39–40.

Jarvis, P. (1992) Reflective practice and nursing. *Nurse Education Today*, **12**, 174–81.

McHaffie, H. (1993) Improving awareness. *Nursing Times*, **89**(18), 29–31.

Newell, R. (1992) Anxiety, accuracy and reflection: the limits of professional development. *Journal of Advanced Nursing*, **17**, 1326–33.

Riverside Health Authority (1990) *HIV, an Ethical Framework*, Riverside Hospitals, London.

Savage, J. (1987) *Nurses, Gender and Sexuality*, Heinemann, London.

Sharp, C., Maychell, K. and Walton, I. (1993) *Nursing and AIDS: Material Matters. Issues, Information and Teaching Materials on HIV and AIDS for Nurses – a Research Study*. National Foundation for Educational Research.

United Kingdom Central Council for Nursing, Midwifery and Health Visiting (1985) *Project 2000: A new preparation for practice*, UKCC, London.

United Kingdom Central Council for Nursing, Midwifery and Health Visiting (1992) *Code of Professional Conduct*, UKCC, London.

United Kingdom Central Council for Nursing, Midwifery and Health Visiting (1993) *Registrar's Letter: Consultation on the Council's Proposed Standards for Post-Registration Education*, UKCC, London.

Wells, R. (1987) *The AIDS Challenge*, Scutari, London.

Wiley, K. and Acklin, M. (1988) Care of AIDS patients: student attitudes. *Nursing Outlook*, **36**, 244–5.

PART TWO
Models, Settings and Responses

INTRODUCTION

This part has been written to provide an insight into how the nursing profession has responded to some of the challenges raised by HIV and AIDS. It explores nursing responses in various settings, e.g. primary and secondary health care, and comments on the basic principles of nursing management. A joint declaration on AIDS from the ICN and WHO highlights the role of the nurse in AIDS care, to the effect that 'the nurse's responsiblity is to those people who require nursing care and that in providing care she/he promotes an environment in which the values, customs and spiritual beliefs of the individual are respected' (ICN/WHO, 1987). WHO has stated that 'no single nursing model or ideal health-care setting can be outlined. Factors that influence the health-care system can include the type of health-care setting, the availability of skilled staff, the technical support available, and the number of patients' (WHO, 1988). The development of appropriate health-care services for people with HIV/AIDS has been greatly influenced over the years by key personnel in the health services. Bennett and Pettigrew (1991) suggest that the 'early movers [in HIV/AIDS], though very different as individual characters, had a common commitment to the cause of HIV/AIDS, an enthusiasm for promoting greater awareness and interest in the issue, and a view of the issue which went beyond the narrow confines of their own specialties. In addition, all displayed a determination to develop the kinds of services they felt appropriate, regardless of even the most protracted opposition'. In many cases, the 'early movers' recognized the vital role people with HIV infection and/or AIDS had in contributing their ideas about developing HIV-related services. Both people with HIV infection and HIV/AIDS non-governmental organizations played an important part in articulating the needs of infected individuals. As a result, it was evident early on that the consultation process could not afford to exclude those who would be using the services. However, in the main this related to the needs of gay men who, through their established networks such as Body Positive, ensured that a 'corporate' voice was heard. As the pandemic continues to change, increasingly health and social care professionals will need to establish services that meet the needs of other client groups, such as women, children, drug users and heterosexual men. Although pioneering groups such as Positively Women, Positive Options and the Black HIV and AIDS Network (BHAN) will continue to represent their clients and attempt to ensure that specific needs are met, the fact that the majority of these groups are located in London and do not have extensive networks throughout the country is cause for concern. Organizations such as Body Positive have, over recent years, opened their doors to all individuals with HIV infection, but anecdotal evidence would suggest that for many people such an organization is not seen as geared up to meet their needs. Service development will continue to be dependent, for the foreseeable future, on the 'product champions', who will be required to push forward the boundaries and ensure that consultation is ongoing.

This next section explores some of the issues raised in developing a range of services in both primary and secondary care settings. It explores and addresses some of the basic principles underpinning service development, provides an insight into philosophies and models of care currently in operation, outlines some of the lessons learnt along the way and describes some of the challenges the nursing profession still faces in developing care options.

REFERENCES

Bennett, C. and Pettigrew, A. (1991) *Pioneering Services for AIDS. The Response to HIV Infection in Four Health Authorities. Final Report,* Centre for Corporate Strategy and Change, University of Warwick.
ICN/WHO (1987) *Joint Declaration on AIDS,* ICN, Geneva.
WHO (1988) *Guidelines for Nursing Management of People Infected with HIV.* WHO AIDS Series No 3. WHO, Geneva.

Primary care and HIV/AIDS **6**

John Hooker

WHAT IS PRIMARY CARE?

Primary health care in the United Kingdom has probably never assumed a position of such importance as it has now. Changes of policy mean that there is increased emphasis, for a variety of reasons, on bringing services out of secondary care and closer to the consumer, i.e. the patient. As primary care assumes new importance, the demands on the service continue to evolve. It has often been said that the single greatest advance in public health was the invention of the water closet in the nineteenth century. Today's health concerns have more complex aetiologies than did cholera and typhoid, and perhaps none pose more intractable problems than does HIV.

The main point of departure between primary and secondary care is that the former normally provides the first point of contact for a person seeking advice, treatment or support. However, for effectiveness, the two parts of the health service must be well integrated. The World Health Organization's elaborate definition of primary care (WHO, 1978) stresses the universality of the availability of the service and the full participation of the community. It further argues that it should foster a 'spirit of self-reliance and self-determination'. Primary care has to encompass not only the care, treatment and rehabilitation of those with acute and chronic illness, but also health promotion and illness prevention. This last hallmark of the WHO definition appears to be particularly apposite for HIV and AIDS. Current trends are moving the service towards an integrated community-based model, such as that developed by Slater (1990), which incorporates all four elements of the WHO philosophy.

PRIMARY CARE IN THE UK

Primary care services in the UK are well developed, with a strong emphasis on the central role of the general medical practitioner and with long-established health visiting and district nursing structures. Nevertheless, despite recent far-reaching changes, primary care is still organized in a relatively complex fashion. Funding derives from the Department of Health and is allocated to the 8 Regional Health Authorities in England. The relevant departments in Northern Ireland, Scotland and Wales similarly fund the health services in those countries (Levitt and Wall, 1992).

In England and Wales there are two types of authority with the ability to commission services. The District Health Authority (DHA) purchases community health services (as well as hospital services) where these have become NHS Trusts. DHAs also manage community services where they have not become Trusts. Family Health Services Authorities (FHSAs) receive funding to allow them to pay for independent practitioner services from the four professions: dentists, general medical practitioners, opticians and pharmacists.

The systems in the two other countries are simpler. Scotland has one authority, the Health Board, which administers all the health services. Within Health Boards, there are Primary Care Divisions which handle the work done by FHSAs in England and Wales. Northern Ireland takes integration a stage further, by having Health and Social Services Boards which manage not only the health functions but also the personal social services. These arrangements are well described by Ham (1991).

UNITARY AUTHORITIES

A further reorganization of health services in England and Wales is under way which will bring them closer to the systems in the rest of the UK. FHSAs and DHAs have for some time been encouraged to work more closely together. Already, consortia of various groupings, the health commissions or commissioning agencies (the titles are as multifarious as the areas they serve), have been formed (Donaldson, 1993). From 1996 it is expected that these new bodies will become unitary authorities once the necessary legislation has been enacted (DoH, 1993a).

The formation of health commissions, with the resulting overview of health provision, should particularly benefit primary care. A 'seamless service' should be achievable if the will is there. More potently, the strategic shift of resources from secondary to primary care should be made easier. This will benefit primary care HIV services, provided that those with the ideas and vision to develop them are able to make their voices heard by the commissioners. Primary care nurses must ensure that the very valuable health needs information around HIV which they acquire is included in the commissioning process.

PURCHASING PRIMARY CARE

The roles of the DHA and FHSA are well described by Ham (1991). Their coming together should make them better at carrying out their health needs assessment and purchasing functions. Although they are still evolving into the authorities of tomorrow, some major trends are already emerging:

- involving local people and organizations, users and carers and clinical staff ('partnership sourcing');
- developing primary care services;
- introducing more quality indicators into contracts, including a greater emphasis on 'charterism';
- commitment to preventive health;
- involving a wider range of people, including nurses, as purchasers.

By simplifying the bureaucracy surrounding health care purchasing, commissions should find it easier to respond to innovative ways of meeting health needs. Nowhere should this be more apparent than in HIV initiatives, which often demand unusual funding arrangements and cross-boundary cooperation, or 'healthy alliances'. Already, examples of imaginative purchasing are beginning to filter through. One such, 'Gay Men Fighting AIDS in London', is funded by eight authorities.

Since their inception, FHSAs have been able to channel funds into specific developments in general practice. Now, with the possibility of funds being switched into primary care, local HIV services at GP level should, in theory at any rate, be increased. Primary care medical advisers and facilitators are well placed to encourage and support GPs and primary care nurses in becoming more involved in caring for people with HIV/AIDS (Layzell and McCarthy, 1992).

Primary care funding also provides for the training of GP practice employed staff, including practice nurses. Commissions and Boards can thus ensure that practice nurses are able to maintain and develop their professional skills, including those concerning HIV, especially prevention.

Commissions and Boards are involved, along with local authorities (except in Northern Ireland, where they are combined) in the community care process which became operative on 1 April 1993. Although local authorities are the lead agencies, the health organizations have major roles in ensuring that the needs of primary care are represented in the process, particularly with respect to discharge arrangements. Purchasing organizations also have to ensure that information is disseminated and education carried out.

The experience from the first year of the new arrangements shows that GPs form the weakest link in the community care chain (King's Fund Centre/Nuffield Institute, 1994). The supplementary, though nonetheless vital, role of GPs and district nurses in assessments, especially joint ones, must be carefully promoted and nurtured (Rom, 1993).

One of the groups for whom authorities have had to draw up plans is precisely people with, or at risk of, HIV/AIDS. Normally, the planning procedure includes consultation. However, this has proved difficult to achieve in the HIV/AIDS field, with clients understandably being unwilling to identify themselves by attending public meetings. The involvement of voluntary organizations has been, in many areas, the only way to ensure that users' views were heard. There is also concern that, in areas of low prevalence, the relevant community care planning groups may disappear altogether, removing at once the focus for local representation and consultation, as has happened with some addiction services. Given the continuously changing nature of the HIV epidemic, the need for well-planned local services remains all the more essential.

GENERAL PRACTICE FUNDHOLDING

A further complication to the primary health care equation is the existence of the GP fundholding scheme, which came into being in April 1991. This allows GPs to hold and manage their own budgets for staffing, training and prescribing, as well as purchasing some types of hospital care on behalf of their patients (Secretaries of State, 1989). From April 1993, the scheme was extended to include certain community services, notably community nursing. Although the spread of fundholding practices is patchy, the numbers are growing steadily every year. In terms of purchasing power, GP fundholders separately have the power to influence the hospital and community care that their patients receive; taken together, their purchasing power will, alongside health commissioning agencies, shape the primary and secondary care of tomorrow.

As purchasers of community nursing, fundholding practices should be able to provide better integrated services to their patients, but there are concerns felt by many nurses over the potential for domination by the medical profession. It is easy to see the possibility of conflicting views arising over the care of people with HIV/AIDS in the community if the GPs feel that the level of care required is taking up a disproportionate amount of district nurse time. Traditionally, access to a district nurse can be obtained without a GP's consent. It will be interesting to note whether community nurse managers will be able to maintain this universality of access within the new arrangements.

One other concern often expressed is over the possible costs of prescribing for people with HIV. However, although fundholders have strictly defined prescribing budgets, there are provisions for regional health authorities to provide extra funding for individual patients whose drug bills are excessive. There should thus be no need for a fundholding practice to remove patients from their list for this reason.

NON-FUNDHOLDING GPS

There are many practices who are, for one reason or another, implacably opposed to fundholding. Nevertheless, some non-fundholding GPs have come to regard fundholders' ability to influence primary and secondary care with more than a hint of jealousy, and their practices have begun seeking similar clout. This is happening in several ways, either through direct input into the health authority's purchasing process, or by the DHA/Health Board setting up some form of practice or locality-sensitive purchasing scheme (GMSC, 1992; Moore, 1993).

CONSUMER ISSUES

The net result of all of this is that the health service is becoming increasingly primary care led. Is it, however, a consumer-led service? In reality, there is not much evidence yet that people with HIV are able to influence the provision of care for themselves. One reason for this lies in the drift of people with HIV, not only from the provinces to the 'centres of excellence', but also from primary to secondary care. Wadsworth and McCann (1992), in a study of gay men with HIV, found 13.3% not registered with a GP. Of those who were registered a significant number had not disclosed their status to their GP, and there was a widespread preference in favour of outpatient clinics rather than GPs for all forms of medical advice. Concerns over the sensitivity of GPs to this and other groups of marginalized patients are confirmed by studies which have looked at GPs' attitudes (Brown-Peterside *et al.*, 1991; Shapiro, 1989).

Anecdotal evidence suggests that people with HIV tend to select a GP by word of mouth recommendation from other people with HIV. One development which has the potential to offer some reassurance to them in making their choice is that of Primary Health Care Charters. While all health authorities have been obliged to draw up Patients' Charters with mandatory standards, primary health care teams are merely to be encouraged by FHSAs/Health Boards to formulate Primary Health Care Charters. By involving the primary health care team in distilling the philosophy and aims of the practice, Charters should include a patient's rights, such as confidentiality, sensitivity to needs and honesty of communication, local standards that the practice or primary health care team has agreed to provide, as well as the expectations of the practice and a 'help us to help you' section (Parr, 1992). Patients should thus be aware of the kind of service they can expect and how to complain if things go wrong. Implicit in the adoption of a Charter is the provision by the practice of some forum for feedback on its services from patients. In areas of high prevalence this would enable people with HIV to have an input into shaping the services available to them. A good example of a Primary Health Care Charter can be found in *General Practitioner* (1993).

PRIMARY HEALTH CARE TEAMS

We must now look at the nuts and bolts of primary care and what it means for HIV and AIDS. The crucial unit for nurses is the primary health care team (PHCT), the basis of which is the GP practice. Successive nursing documents, from the Cumberlege Report (HMSO, 1986) to *New World, New Opportunities* (NHSME, 1993), have reaffirmed this position. GP practices are therefore the *locus operandi* for most primary care nurses.

The extension of the GP fundholding scheme to include community services from 1 April 1993 may well help to strengthen the medical leadership of the PHCT. However, success depends to a large extent on there being a 'benevolent dictatorship'. Dominance by one professional grouping works against cooperation and can suppress the potential of other team members, most of whom are nurses.

Given that empowerment of the individual forms a major part of the philosophy of HIV care, a conflicting ethos affecting primary care workers does not bode well for the care they are able to provide. Similarly, a medical model of care can work against empowerment. By contrast, nursing models such as Orem's self-care model are well suited for nurses seeking to enable individuals to increase control over their illness and care, besides which these models are particularly appropriate in HIV work, especially from a health promotion viewpoint (Hartweg, 1990).

To be effective, primary care nurses must seek partnerships within the PHCT and promote their own role and potential. More importantly, the team must also be outward looking in developing alliances with outside groups and individuals. This is crucial in HIV work since, to have maximum effect, prevention has to work at a number of levels, and care of those affected demands input by a number of agencies, both professional and lay.

Although the composition of the PHCT has almost as many variants as there are writers on the subject, current thinking, as exemplified by Marsh (1993), suggests the following groups:

- reception, records and computer staff;
- office and administrative staff;
- the nursing team;
- other professional advisers (social worker, physiotherapist, dietitian etc.);
- the doctors;
- occasional members of the team (accountants, ministers of religion etc.);
- missing people such as chiropodists, complementary therapists, dentists etc.

For the person with HIV every one of these groups has potential importance. A growing number of practices, mostly fundholders, are able to offer a counsellor or complementary therapist. Anecdotally, there are a few practices currently able to offer dedicated counselling services to their seropositive patients, but developments such as this require extra funding from FHSAs.

Those at risk of HIV may also need the services of the PHCT. In reality, GPs and primary care nurses are the most important members of the team as far as prevention is concerned. Nevertheless, others might also have important roles to play. Receptionists, for example, are extremely important as portals of access to other team members. Receptionists' attitudes towards known HIV patients led to reports of some horrifying incidents in the early days of the epidemic. The manner of the receptionist might be an important factor in determining whether a patient feels comfortable in, say, requesting a supply of free condoms.

PHCTs have the potential to provide services at all stages of HIV infection. They also play an increasingly vital role in prevention, as well as in testing. They can also provide important links with community-based groups and have the potential for developing outreach.

THE PHCT AND CARE

GPs have roles in prevention, diagnosis, referral and treatment. Lack of time often precludes their becoming involved extensively in support and counselling. Nevertheless, GPs who feel well disposed towards caring for patients with HIV are able to provide good, and often innovative, services. A survey by Roderick *et al.* (1990) found great potential for the involvement of GPs in caring for people with HIV, but a major limiting factor was the lack of preparation. In addition, there were worries expressed by GUM consultants about issues of confidentiality in general practice. There was most support for a system of shared care. To some extent this is becoming the pattern in some areas of high prevalence. It is possible to see increased pressure for this to be so, given that, as a result of the Tomlinson Report, the number of hospital beds in London is to be reduced (Cruickshanks, 1993).

The improvements required to enable good-quality care for people with HIV within general practice are being sought in a number of ways. Several FHSAs, about 10 at the latest count, have appointed primary care facilitators for HIV/AIDS and a number of other facilitators have HIV/AIDS as a major component of their work. These work mainly, though not exclusively, in large cities: Edinburgh, Leeds, London, Manchester etc. Luff (1991) describes the work of a specialist facilitator in Sheffield who carried out in-depth work with PHCTs, including tailor-made training. This work involved clients in defining the training needs of their practice.

Training for PHCTs has to encompass the triad of knowledge, skills and attitudes. The last of these is perhaps the most resistant to change and there is much to be tackled, given the opinions revealed by significant numbers of both nurses (Bond *et al.*, 1990) and doctors (Brown-Peterside *et al.*, 1991). If there were to be an attitudinal change in the 20% of the GPs surveyed by Brown-Peterside *et al.* (1991) who were unwilling to accept high-risk patients, much could be achieved. Overcoming prejudice against groups already marginalized by society which means poorer services for members of those groups, whether they have HIV or not, must be a prime aim of education. It is possible that this may be partly tackled through the normalization of HIV. This strengthens the argument for normalizing HIV training within a general sexual health context.

Luff (1993) provides a cogent case for the role of the primary care facilitator for HIV/AIDS. However, encouraging PHCTs to recognize that they have a crucial and often unrecognized role to play in HIV prevention and care is not exclusive to specialist facilitators. Many of the over 200 generic primary care facilitators, as well as health education/promotion officers and district HIV prevention coordinators are also involved in education of PHCT members around these issues.

A model of good practice is offered by the Foundation for AIDS Counselling Treatment and Support (FACTS) in North London (Gibbon, 1993; Layzell and McCarthy, 1992). This began as a specialized branch of a general practice, but is now a registered charity with a complex funding arrangement. FACTS offers to share the burden of caring for a person with HIV or AIDS with their GP. As well as mainstream treatments and support, FACTS offers its clients several complementary therapies which are particularly popular. However, one of the main aims of FACTS is to encourage GPs to become more involved in care. To this end, FACTS has invested heavily in education to enable GPs to be able to look after well HIV patients throughout their illness.

One big stumbling block that prevents more GPs from taking on larger portions of care is funding. Although clinics receive extra funding for looking after HIV patients, GPs do not. This is an anomaly which must be addressed if a shift from secondary to primary care is to be accomplished.

The contribution of nurses in primary care is extremely important. Discussion of the role of district nurses in the community care of people with HIV or AIDS is found in Chapter 7. However, it is indeed worrying that, in a 1988 survey, over a third of nurses still wanted to be able to refuse to nurse a patient with HIV (Bond *et al.*, 1990). These researchers found a significant minority of community nurses with negative beliefs about patients with AIDS, and this finding was echoed by the research of Akinsanya and Rouse (1992) with hospital nurses. Cole and Slocumb (1993) found that, like doctors, nurses' attitudes towards patients with AIDS were 'influenced by the mode of acquiring the virus', with more blame being attached to gay men and drug users. This problem has been tackled by many authorities as one of a lack of knowledge. Some are also developing more specific initiatives to overcome these attitude problems.

Community psychiatric nurses (CPNs) have the potential for a major involvement in care of people with HIV-related dementia. A good example of this is the Worcester Development Project, which provides access to a CPN for all people with the virus. The basis of the success of this scheme is the good integration of the CPNs into the PHCT (Bennett,

1989). There is also the potential for involvement with specific individuals. Ronald et al. (1992) describe the work of a CPN in an Edinburgh practice with a large number of infected intravenous drug users.

In contrast, the focus of health visitors and school nurses is largely one of prevention. Practice nurses are also ideally placed to carry out preventive work and may also be involved in some testing. Their role in caring for seropositive patients is coming to the fore in areas of high prevalence (Ronald *et al.*, 1992). The practice nurse's importance lies in his or her accessibility, being often the first point of contact for the patient with the practice. Within her integrated community-based care model for infected individuals, Slater (1990) sees practice nurses being able to provide listening and counselling. However, given the longer survival rates, the practice nurse should be able to address quality of life issues and to assist in rehabilitation within a multidisciplinary approach (Lang, 1993; Wells, 1993). Rehabilitation should encompass preventive, restorative, supportive and palliative stages. Practice nurses and others involved in care can offer much in all of these stages. As Wells (1993) eloquently put it: 'Rehabilitation must in the future form the basis of an holistic approach to the needs of people with AIDS'.

The potential for practice nurses in care of the HIV patient is great, but at present largely untapped. Besides listening and counselling, the practice nurse can use his or her skills in health promotion to help the patient achieve lifestyle changes to maximize health. These include stressing the benefit to the immune system of exercise, relaxation and avoiding stressors and toxins such as tobacco and alcohol, harm reduction for intravenous drug users and safer sex. They can also act as a repository of information about community-based groups such as ACET and home-support teams. They can also provide support, advice and teaching about infection control matters to partners and carers. Again, this might include advice on safer sex.

Many nurses have demonstrated an aptitude for and interest in complementary therapies. These have proved particularly acceptable to people with HIV, and could be included in the service offered by practice nurses. Mainstream treatments, such as i.v. gancyclovir and inhaled pentamidine could be provided for mobile patients unable to have them at home for one reason or another. All these services could be offered in dedicated nurse-run clinics or via open access.

THE PHCT AND TESTING

The role of practice nurses in testing is one which concerns. As employees of GPs, all too often tasks like this are delegated to them. In a survey of GPs, Hoolaghan *et al.* (1993) found that 1% never counsel a patient before testing for HIV, and 10% only counsel 'sometimes'. In a situation such as this, the nurse will have to be able to assure him or herself that the patient is giving specific informed consent for the test. The UKCC (1994) is unequivocal about the fact that nurses lay themselves open to charges of assault if they cooperate in taking blood specimens without consent. Even when they have established that the patient has consented to have blood tested for HIV, they must also establish that proper pretest counselling has been given. If they fail to do this, they could be contravening the UKCC Code of Professional Conduct.

If the nurse is completing the test, he or she should ensure that the patient is aware of confidentiality issues. This should include some discussion of the potential effects on the individual of simply having a test, and the implications of having this recorded in their medical records. They should always offer to send off the test under a code, such as 'Soundex' (Pidcock, 1992, Appendix 2).*

There is little evidence to show that HIV testing is effective as a specific prevention measure. In a review of the evidence to date, Beardsell (1994) found that there is 'insufficient empirical evidence for a clear statement on the effects of testing and counselling'. Nevertheless, despite doubts about effectiveness, the opportunity for discussing prevention issues should not be missed. The occasion of submitting themselves for a test is obviously an extremely important one for the individual. They may well be in a heightened emotional state, which the nurse should be aware of. People will respond to such a situation in different ways, some being more receptive to information and others less so. The nurse will therefore have to carefully assess the need for further counselling.

THE PHCT AND PREVENTION

One of the major planks in the UK Government's response to HIV is that of prevention. HIV/AIDS and sexual health was chosen as one of the five key target areas of the *Health of the Nation* White Paper (DoH, 1992). The specific targets are:

*Unlike GUM clinics, GP practices are not obliged to maintain anonymity. Practice nurses should ensure that issues of anonymity in testing and other confidentiality questions are discussed by the PHCT and that protocols are developed.

- to reduce the incidence of gonorrhoea (as a vector for HIV) among men and women aged 15–64 by at least 20% by 1995;
- to reduce the rate of conceptions among the under 16s by at least 50% by the year 2000;
- to reduce the percentage of injecting drug misusers who report sharing injecting equipment in the previous 4 weeks by at least 50% by 1997, and by at least a further 50% by the year 2000.

Thus the challenge for primary care is explicit, and it is in a good position to respond. The UK's primary health system benefits from having a live register of patients. Taken together with the computerization of many GP practices, particularly fundholders, and the health needs information now available from health authorities, more information is available to practices for planning their services than ever before. On the down side, while they support the targets many health professionals question whether they can be met (George, 1992).

Around 90% of all patient contact with health services occurs in primary care. It has been estimated that in any one year 66% of the population consults their GP, and that in a 5-year period at least 90% will do so. Thus primary care has the ability to reach most of the public. Is it possible, however, in the limited contact time available, to convey meaningful health messages about HIV, along with all the other *Health of the Nation* target areas? The answer has to be that, while posters, leaflets and other displays, particularly if used in concert with specific events such as World AIDS Day, may have some impact, a much more focused approach is required. In addition, as Lucas (1992) puts it, there is a need for the creation of a local healthy alliance within the overall lead from the health authority. Encouragement and support for primary care prevention initiatives will clearly come from the District HIV Prevention Coordinator, with further help from facilitators where available.

What types of HIV prevention activity are being developed in primary care? As a follow-up to the White Paper, the Department of Health (1993b) has produced a comprehensive handbook for HIV/AIDS and sexual health. This contains many examples of local initiatives, much of which invoke the spirit of the healthy alliance. Readers are strongly recommended to seek out this helpful publication, which is also available on disk to achieve maximum impact.

Many GP practices are now offering family planning services. This often involves practice nurses, most of whom will now have had access to specific training. Family planning offers unique possibilities for discussing sexual matters, and every patient should have the opportunity to discuss HIV in relation to themselves. A major problem lies in reaching young people, but many nurses are reluctant to give information and advice to young people even though the 'Gillick' ruling allows that any competent young person, irrespective of age, can seek medical advice and give consent to treatment.

Some practices have partially circumvented the problem of attracting young people by offering Well Teenager Clinics, which are advertised as being for general health matters for the over-16s. The subtext of such clinics is that the attender will be given the chance to discuss HIV prevention issues, along with other risk-taking behaviours. However, developments along these lines can only form part of the picture. As Bury (1991) puts it: 'There is ample evidence that the simple provision of factual information is not sufficient to change behaviour....Young people need to have the opportunity to discuss in small groups the issues raised, so that they can clarify their own values and attitudes....' A range of initiatives aimed at young people is thus necessary. Sex education is a major concern, though often hamstrung by the restrictions that can be imposed by school governors. Where possible, school nurses should become involved in school-based HIV prevention education. In addition, there needs to be peer education and other projects through youth clubs etc., particularly focusing on increasing assertiveness in young women (Jackson, 1991).

Most travellers will attend their local practice for travel immunizations. Again, this is an opportunity for practice nurses to reinforce advice on safer sex while on holiday or business trips. Where the practice is able to offer supplies of free condoms, these can be offered to the traveller.

Many districts have introduced free condom schemes in general practice and these have been carefully evaluated. Although uptake has been good, doubts have been expressed over the effectiveness of the schemes in reaching those most at risk. Many of the condoms distributed appear to have been intended for use largely as a contraceptive measure. However, a trial in Oxford (Pengilley and Kay, 1992) found good uptake from the student population as an HIV prevention measure. There is obviously a need for careful planning and marketing of such a service.

Jackson (1991) believes that health visitors should use every opportunity to discuss HIV/AIDS. By definition, the bulk of their clients are, or have recently been, sexually active. Working with young women with whom they have close relationships should enable them to introduce the subject at the client's own pace. Nevertheless, health visitors are increasingly moving away from devoting most of their time to the 0–5-year-olds to a wider public health role. Fundholding practices are often keen for health visitors to take part in practice-based health promotion activities. This may include the types of HIV prevention work described above involving practice nurses. Besides this, by virtue of their training and experience they may be able to undertake group work. In addition, there is tremendous scope for outreach into the community. Cameron *et al.* (1993) describe the work of a group of health visitors in an outreach project in Edinburgh aimed at providing friendship, support and counselling to sex workers.

A group of primary care nurses that could be overlooked are occupational health nurses. These also provide a service to large numbers of people who are likely to be sexually active. They usually hold a position of trust with employees and their advice is valued. They are thus well placed to give information on safer sex. They should also be alert to the possibility of employees using drugs. Again, most employees will take holidays and managers will often have business trips abroad, and the nurse can reinforce travel advice, including the need for safer sex. In multinational companies, employees going to work abroad, particularly in countries such as the United States, may be required to undergo an HIV antibody test. The nurse may have to deal with the issues around testing, including using this occasion as an opportunity for giving HIV prevention counselling (McGurk, 1991).

CONCLUSION

The restructuring of the health service in the United Kingdom has created a more flexible system. Although the organization of primary care is still relatively complex, there appears to be considerable scope, within the new arrangements being currently developed, for imaginative commissioning and financing of primary care HIV services. Primary care must be in the vanguard of developing innovative and patient-centred services for those already infected with HIV, and has a particularly vital role to play in prevention. Nurses working in this field must work along with their colleagues in primary care and others in their locality so that they can help build services to match local needs.

HIV is everyone's problem. The message of *The Health of the Nation* is that all nurses working in primary care have a duty to respond to the challenge in whatever way they can. By forging healthy alliances across boundaries, with local authority workers, the voluntary sector, schools and colleges, patients and clients themselves, and working together as fully fledged and committed primary health care teams, primary care nurses can make a substantial contribution in prevention, in dealing with issues around testing and in the care of those infected with, and affected by, the virus.

REFERENCES

Akinsanya, J. A. and Rouse, P. (1992) Who will care? A survey of the knowledge and attitudes of hospital nurses to people with HIV/AIDS. *Journal of Advanced Nursing*, **17**, 400–1.

Beardsell, S. (1994) Should wider HIV testing be encouraged on the grounds of HIV prevention? *AIDS Care*, **6**(1), 5–19.

Bennett, C. (1989) The Worcester Development Project: general practitioner satisfaction with a new community psychiatric service. *Journal of the Royal College of General Practitioners*, **39**, 106–9.

Bond, S., Rhodes, T., Philips, P. and Tierney, A. (1990) HIV infection and community nursing staff in Scotland – 2: Knowledge and attitudes. (Occasional Paper.) *Nursing Times*, **86**(45), 49–51.

Brown-Peterside, P., Sibbald, B. and Freeling, P. (1991) AIDS: Knowledge, skills and attitudes among vocational trainees and their trainers. *British Journal of General Practice*, **41**, 401–5.

Bury, J. K. (1991) Teenage sexual behaviour and the impact of AIDS. *Health Education Journal*, **50**(1), 43–9.

Cameron, S., Peacock, W. and Trotter, G. (1993) Reaching out. *Nursing Times*, **89**(7), 34–6.

Cole, F.L. and Slocumb, E.M. (1993) Nurses' attitudes toward patients with AIDS. *Journal of Advanced Nursing*, **18**, 1112–17.

Cruickshanks, M. (1993) Nurses remain ignorant over HIV/AIDS. *British Journal of Nursing*, **2**(4), 207.

Department of Health (1992) *The Health of the Nation: A Strategy for Health in England*, HMSO, London.

Department of Health (1993a) *Managing the New NHS*, Department of Health, Leeds.

Department of Health (1993b) *The Health of the Nation. Key Area Handbook. HIV/AIDS and Sexual Health*, Department of Health, London.

Donaldson, L. (1993) The primary aim is to give patients better care. *The Independent*, 20 May 1993.

General Medical Services Committee (1992) *Commissioning Care: Options for GPs*, BMA, London.

General Practitioner (1993) Guide: Primary healthcare charter. *General Practitioner*, 15 January, 71–4.

George, M. (1992) Aiming too high? *Nursing Standard*, **6**(48), 20–1.

Gibbon, J. (1993) Teaching the facts about AIDS. *The Independent*, 17 June.

Ham, C. (1991) *The New National Health Service Organization and Management*, Radcliffe Medical Press, Oxford.

Hartweg, D. L. (1990) Health promotion self-care within Orem's general theory of nursing. *Journal of Advanced Nursing*, **15**, 35–41.

Her Majesty's Stationery Office (1986) *Neighbourhood Nursing – A Focus for Care*, HMSO, London.

Hoolaghan, T., Blache, G. and Pidcock, J. (1993) *The Role of General Practitioners in HIV Prevention: Findings from a Questionnaire Survey*, Camden and Islington Health Promotion Service, London.

Jackson, C. (1991) Getting the message across. *Health Visitor*, **64**(7), 212–13.

King's Fund Centre/Nuffield Institute (1994) *Fit for Change? Snapshots of the Community Care Reforms One Year On*, King's Fund Centre/Nuffield Institute, London.

Lang, C. (1993) Positive steps. *Nursing Times*, **89**(11), 54–6.

Layzell, S. and McCarthy, M. (1992) Developing services for people with HIV/AIDS: The role of FHSAs. *Primary Health Care Management*, **2**(13), 2–4.

Levitt, R. and Wall, A. (1992) *The Reorganized National Health Service*, 4th edn, Chapman & Hall, London.

Lucas, G. (1992) Responding to *Health of the Nation* targets for HIV/AIDS and sexual health, in *HIV Prevention. A Working Guide for Professionals*, (ed. P. Jones), Health Education Authority, London, p.17.

Luff, D. (1991) General practice and HIV – in need of a facilitator? *Health Education Journal*, **50**(3), 146–8.

Luff, D. (1993) An HIV facilitator in general practice. *British Journal of Sexual Medicine*, Jan/Feb, 4–6.

McGurk, M. D. (1991) AIDS and the international traveller: 2. *Occupational Health*, March, 74–80.

Marsh, G. (1993) Achieving the full potential of the primary health care team. *Primary Health Care Management*, **3**(1), 5–7.

Moore, W. (1993) Commissioning healthcare: the GP's choice. *Management in General Practice*, **7**, 18-21.

National Health Service Management Executive (1993) *New World, New Opportunities*, HMSO, London.

Parr, C. (1992) The Patient's Charter and primary care. *Management in General Practice*, **6**, 14–15.

Pengilley, L. and Kay, R. (1992) *Condom Study. October–December 1991*, Oxfordshire Family Health Service Authority, Oxford.

Pidcock, J. (1992) *Conference Report 'The Role of General Practitioners in HIV Prevention'*, Camden and Islington Health Promotion Service, London.

Roderick, P., Victor, C. R. and Beardow, R. (1990) Developing care in the community: GPs and the HIV epidemic. *AIDS Care*, **2**(2), 127–32.

Rom, J. (1993) Community care: making assessment worthwhile. *Primary Health Care Management*, **3**(1), 8–9.

Ronald, P. J. M., Witcomb, J. C., Robertson, J. R. *et al.* (1992) Problems of drug abuse, HIV and AIDS: the burden of care in one general practice. *British Journal of General Practice*, **42**, 232–5.

Secretaries of State for Health, Wales, Northern Ireland and Scotland (1989) *Working for Patients*, HMSO, London.

Shapiro, J. A. (1989) General practitioners' attitudes towards AIDS and their perceived information needs. *British Medical Journal*, **298**, 1563–6.

Slater, C. (1990) An integrated approach to HIV and AIDS. *Practice Nurse*, June, 75–8.

United Kingdom Central Council for Nurses, Midwives and Health Visitors (1994) Registrar's Letter 4/1994 Annexe 1. UKCC, London.

Wadsworth, E. and McCann, K. (1992) Attitudes towards and use of general practitioner services among homosexual men with HIV infection or AIDS. *British Journal of General Practice*, **42**, 107–10.

Wells, R. (1993) The rehabilitation of people with AIDS. *Nursing Standard*, **7**(25), 51–3.

World Health Organization (1978) *Primary Health Care*. Report of the International Conference on Primary Health Care, Alma Ata, USSR 6–12 September 1978. World Health Organization, Geneva.

Community nursing and HIV – challenging the system

7

Neil Brocklehurst and Geraldine Reilly

INTRODUCTION

A recurrent theme in this book is the relationship between specialist and generalist nurses in the field of HIV health care. Nowhere has this issue been more passionately debated than in the context of community nursing.

Early in the epidemic, when comparatively little was known about the disease, the most effective response to care came from a small group of 'product champions' (Bennett and Pettigrew, 1991). These dedicated practitioners were willing to take up the challenges posed by this stigmatizing illness. The hospital focus was inevitable, considering the need for intensive and unusual treatments required by those presenting with symptoms. Consequently, hospital-based specialist outreach teams developed, providing nursing and medical care across the divide between hospital and community.

A series of hospital and community nursing research studies indicated that substantial numbers of generic nurses felt unprepared and often unwilling to care for people with HIV disease (Akinsanya and Rouse, 1991; Bond et al., 1991; Bond and Rhodes, 1990; Tierney et al., 1990). Against this background, it was easy to understand why many individuals opted to stay with a specialist service that was seen as knowledgeable and non-judgemental. However, some providers who foresaw the rise in numbers needing care, soon realized that continuing to develop a separate service would be financially unviable and even undesirable, since it emphasized the isolation of a group already viewed as unpopular by health-care staff (Wolf, 1989).

The specialist vs. generic debate was set within the context of a rapidly changing health-care system, concerned with value for money, internal markets and increasing attention on the community as the main focus of care. Thus, alongside a number of pressing practical issues linked to the fact that people lived longer with an incurable disease, policy matters also had to be addressed.

The timing of the HIV epidemic has therefore been very interesting, and the concern generated by it has forced us to look again, albeit from a rather different angle, at some of the most important aspects of community nursing care:

- shared care;
- discharge planning;
- home care and the involvement of informal carers.

This chapter addresses these issues, highlighting the state of the art in nursing research and practice and indicating some of the important implications that HIV has created for policy.

SHARED CARE

HIV disease is now understood to manifest itself as a chronic, progressive illness, commonly comprising a lengthy period of wellness followed by increasingly frequent, though irregular, episodes of acute infection. For this reason alone, most peoples' needs will change over time. Early diagnosis affords the opportunity to assess a person's health at regular intervals, while late stage disease often requires multiple hospital episodes, ongoing intravenous therapy to combat opportunistic infection and symptom control.

The range of needs highlighted above indicates important roles for hospital specialists, palliative care teams, the district nurse and the general practitioner. At its best, the health service can provide a combination of expertise, home care and effective teamwork. Shared care, a concept familiar to anyone involved in the maternity services, offers a framework for a comprehensive health and social care package to anyone affected by HIV.

Shared care in HIV must involve the hospital, the community services and the client. In addition, it may also need to involve one or more informal carer (e.g. parent, partner or sibling). To be effective, the content and delivery of shared care needs to be agreed by all those involved, roles must be clearly defined and respected, and care should be characterized by high-quality communication, however exacting these requirements may be.

In a recent study examining continuity of care for people with HIV disease (Brocklehurst *et al.*, 1993), shared care protocols were found to be rarely in evidence, with general practitioners seldom actively involved in care and community nurses mainly utilized in the later stages of the disease process, suggesting several major barriers to shared care. Good practice, however, was being pursued and developed in some areas, with hospital liaison teams vigorously engaging in a strategy of early primary care involvement. In these cases, and a number of others, the presence of link persons between hospital and community proves vital, although these may not always need to possess a nursing or medical background (Smith *et al.*, 1993).

Another crucial element of successful shared care is the active participation of the GP, but progress in this area has been slow. In a recently published report concerning HIV-positive clients' contacts with services (Hull–York Research Team, 1993), it was found that although the majority of people studied were registered with a GP, a quarter had changed their GP since diagnosis and a third said their GP was unaware of their HIV status. These findings reflect earlier work indicating that family doctors have been reluctant to care for people with the virus, particularly drug users (Foy and Gallagher, 1990).

General lack of knowledge of the disease process on the part of GPs also explains why people affected by the virus have been slow to use primary health services. This has been in part attributable to the widespread availability of primary care offered by specialist outpatient departments. High staff turnover in such units, together with a frequent lack of training and experience of general health care, may be preventing patients from receiving the best primary medical care. General practitioners must be encouraged to share their expertise, both with specialist units and with HIV-positive patients.

In view of the ability of fundholding GPs to purchase community nursing and hospital care for their patients, they have to understand the existence and needs of the HIV-positive population that they serve. Specialist units in some areas are now encouraging GPs to participate in care, through the provision of accredited courses, improved communication and shared care protocols. Both clinical nurse specialists in HIV and hospital physicians have important roles to play in promoting greater levels of shared care.

Client-held records, specifying such things as treatment regimens, up-to-date blood test results and key contacts, are an obvious and effective means of conveying important information in a confidential manner, but there is little evidence from current HIV-related literature to suggest that their use is widespread. Success in the use of such records in child and maternal health care indicates that greater attention should be paid to its development in the field of HIV.

It is clear, therefore, that the debate about specialist and generic services cannot be seen in either/or terms. Both have important roles to play in the provision of continuing care to people with HIV disease, and many models already exist elsewhere in the health-care system. It may appear that their incorporation into HIV care has been slow, but this generally occurs in units which remain isolated from other hospital departments and the community.

DISCHARGE PLANNING

Many issues relevant to shared care arise during discharge planning for people due to be released from hospital.

Preparation of patients for discharge from hospital has been given widespread attention by researchers (Waters, 1987; Jowett and Armitage, 1988; Singleton, 1990) and policy makers (DH, 1989a), and the complexities of HIV care have once more highlighted the importance of effective planning.

In their large-scale study in Wales, Armitage and colleagues concluded that liaison between hospital and community staff was a vital part of the discharge process and they identified three different models of liaison:

1. Direct liaison between ward staff in community hospitals and community nursing staff, without an intermediary.
2. Direct liaison between nurses in district general hospitals and the community, without an intermediary.
3. Indirect liaison between nurses in district general hospitals and the community, with the help of a liaison nurse.

They found that the most effective communication occurred in model one and the most ineffective in model two, reflecting the (increasing) distance between hospital and community staff in large urban areas (Armitage and Jowett, 1988).

Given that most hospital care for people with HIV disease takes place in large teaching hospitals, there should be no surprise in research findings indicating that the most effective discharge planning and liaison occurs where a liaison team (with district nursing experience) acts as an intermediary between hospital and community (Brocklehurst et al., 1993). The effectiveness of model one outlined above does highlight the fact, however, that direct nurse-to-nurse communication should be promoted at all times. Hospital liaison teams operate best and are most widely accepted when they facilitate ward nurses in their work rather than taking over referrals and discharge planning completely.

A number of important points in hospital discharge for people with HIV require consideration:

1. Effective planning can only occur with the involvement of the multidisciplinary team, including the patient and any chosen informal carers.
2. Clarity of roles among the planning team is required, particularly during the assessment phase, when liaison staff, ward nurses, care managers and other therapy staff may all wish to interview the patient and be involved in home visits.
3. Ward charge nurses must ensure that their staff are aware of local admission and discharge policies. Where these are inappropriate in relation to HIV (e.g. regarding confidentiality), they must ensure that policies are updated and widely publicized.
4. Community services already engaged in a patient's care should be informed of hospital admission within 24 hours of its occurrence.
5. Discharge planning should start at the time of admission, anticipating treatment, length of stay, place of discharge and the care needed on discharge. The patient's consent must be obtained before services are involved.
6. Wherever possible, the relevant services should have 7 days' notice of discharge. This enables community carers to meet the patient prior to discharge (something to be strongly encouraged) and to arrange for any equipment or medications to be ordered in advance.
7. Patients being transferred to convalescent units must be assured of a hospital bed should readmission be required.
8. Appropriate accommodation for those in later-stage illness needs to be planned in advance. Occupational therapy home assessments can be invaluable in such circumstances, and mechanisms for joint working with relevant housing authorities or associations must be set up well in advance of need.

Our experience has shown that weekly multidisciplinary meetings designed to discuss each patient's discharge arrangements are important in forward planning and provide an excellent opportunity for all members of the team to meet. Where a patient's needs are particularly complex, case conferences provide the most effective means of planning care, but careful thought must be given to the best way of involving a patient who may be severely ill and unable to communicate their wishes easily.

It is impossible to be prescriptive about each individual's roles in the discharge process, since much will depend on the relationships established with any particular patient. As mentioned above, role clarity is essential to successful discharge planning and time needs to be taken by the care team to create a framework for joint working. Such a framework should stress patient centrality, acknowledge individual practitioners' knowledge and skills and facilitate effective communication among the team.

Ultimately, the outcome of discharge will indicate the ability of the team to manage the process successfully, and it is therefore important to devise methods of evaluating discharge. Lessons can be learned from the approach taken by researchers investigating this area of care: common features of the work carried out by those mentioned in this section include direct observation of ward staff, examination of hospital records and patient interviews. If greater attention was routinely paid to these aspects of discharge, it is likely that documentation and record keeping would improve and all staff would benefit from a deeper understanding of the whole process of hospital discharge.

DISTRICT NURSING AND HOME CARE

For the majority of patients discharged from hospital, including those with HIV disease, the result is a return home. For patients in late-stage illness, there is often a need for ongoing community care.

In the introduction to this chapter we explored the development of specialist home care teams in HIV and discussed the problems associated with involving the community care team. It has been interesting to chart the progress of some of the specialist teams, most of which are to be found in London. In virtually all cases there has been much greater integration of these teams into existing generic services, frequently in an effort to contain costs and avoid service duplication.

Despite earlier findings suggesting some unwillingness to provide care to people with HIV disease, the most recent comprehensive study looking at the role of the district nurse indicates a strong commitment by generic nurses to this client group (Brocklehurst *et al.*, 1993).

In view of these findings, and in the light of experience, we are in favour of a model of community nursing that involves both generic and specialist staff. District nurses have shown themselves willing to care for people with HIV, provided they have open access to specialist knowledge and advice, are fully supported by their local managers and given adequate supervision on a regular basis.

Hospitals should thus provide link liaison nurses who are fully aware of both community and hospital policies. These must work with the primary health-care team (PHCT) in establishing communication channels, providing support, education and training, and developing shared care protocols. It is important that community nurses do not feel isolated in their work with HIV patients, especially as clinical nurse specialists in HIV have proved popular with their generic colleagues (Haste and Macdonald, 1992). All district nurses caring for people with HIV disease should be able to administer therapy intravenously. Although access to training has been problematic in some areas, we have not encountered any insurmountable barriers to this problem. Regular updating is important and provides another reason for greater collaboration between hospital and community nurses.

The majority of contact with community nurses for people with HIV disease has so far been with district nurses, reflecting the late stage in illness at which the service tends to be involved. As the epidemic continues to spread among different groups in the population, and the progress towards cure remains painfully slow, health visitors, community midwives, community psychiatric and other nurses working outside hospitals must become more involved.

Locally based community practitioners are best placed, not only to provide specialist medical and nursing care, but also to promote sexual health and prevent unnecessary illness. These practitioners must provide support and advice to those perceiving themselves to be at risk as well as those already affected by the disease. To do so effectively, they must have access to the education and training discussed by Carol Pellowe in Chapter 5.

TERMINAL CARE

In the previous section we considered the issue of maintaining good health for both HIV-positive and HIV-negative people. In both the lay and the professional community the emphasis has been on 'living with AIDS'. What does this mean for those who have to die with AIDS?

One of the main and continuing problems associated with palliative care in HIV disease has been the difficulty in defining 'end stage'. We have frequently experienced patients who, against all expectation, return to work after a particularly serious opportunistic infection. In addition, the interface between curative and palliative treatments, whereby active investigations and new drug trials appear to go hand in hand with advice on symptom control, further confuses the problem of defining the various stages of the disease.

Given the unpredictable period of later-stage illness, it is important that patients are able to spend time in the care setting of their choice. For most, this will be their own home. The PHCT and the individual affected need to know each other prior to this time. Only in these circumstances can patients and their carer(s) be supported and enabled to make informed decisions regarding the final phase of their life.

Crucial medical decisions near the time of death need to be taken in the context of a thorough appraisal of the person's situation. For example, the question of whether or not to continue with intravenous therapy to prevent blindness in the final weeks of life needs to be addressed in the context of the total number of drugs being taken and the overall quality of life. If patients live far from their treatment centre or are too unwell to attend, the primary care teams are best placed to help answer these questions. If the local primary care team is involved only at the terminal stage, it is unlikely that adequate or satisfactory answers can be found.

Options for respite and terminal HIV care vary according to geographical location. In London, for example, HIV-specific facilities now exist for children, families, people with drug problems and those with severe brain impairment. These services have been widely used and have affected the place of death for patients in that area (Quirk and Reilly, 1993). Elsewhere there remains little choice other than traditional hospices, an increasing number of which are offering services to people with HIV disease (Shailer *et al.*, 1993). However, the age, complex therapeutic requirements and lifestyles of some affected individuals indicate that a wider range of options is needed.

Specialist nursing services, such as Marie Curie and Macmillan teams, have developed a range of skills that can greatly benefit those with HIV disease, yet there appears to be little involvement by these providers to date, with attention focusing more on diagnosis (e.g. cancer) than need. As in other areas of health care, HIV has focused attention on the wider problem facing those with palliative and terminal care needs who do not fall into any particular disease category. It has delivered a timely reminder of the need for a wider review of palliative care, in both hospital and the community.

INVOLVING INFORMAL CARERS

The contribution to long-term community care made by informal carers has long been recognized by social scientists, and recently in policy, with the provision of care managers for carers within the NHS and Community Care Act (1990) legislation.

Community nurses, in our experience, have often registered surprise at the level of care provided by partners of people with HIV disease. For many professionals it will be the first time that they have had any close contact with the gay community or encountered significant numbers of young male carers. Additionally, there are few other diseases where carers may themselves be infected and may follow a course of illness similar to those they care for.

The level of support and practical help needed by informal carers should not be underestimated. Interestingly, in the study mentioned previously (Brocklehurst *et al.*, 1993) it was found that district nurses described listening and talking to carers as one of their most time-consuming tasks with the client group.

Carers may feel isolated if assessments and plans exclude their contribution to care, and they may feel alienated if their own specific needs are not taken into consideration by the care team. The primary care team has an important role to play in including carers in decisions, thus providing further justification for early team involvement: the longer time this affords for developing relationships with both patient and carer should enable decisions regarding treatment and continuing care to be tailored to individual needs.

Although professionals frequently describe the difficulties associated with maintaining high levels of confidentiality with patients with HIV disease, carers often have a far greater burden to carry, fending off inquisitive relatives for months or even years on end. Thus not only should they have access to accurate information about respite facilities, welfare benefits and home care, they also need to be offered time and space to voice their frustrations and worries. It is likely that well-supported community nurses are best equipped to identify carers' emotional needs and provide the most appropriate response.

It is therefore apparent that carers' and patients' needs do not always coincide, and that professionals may be called on to arbitrate and negotiate when conflicts arise. The advent of recent community care legislation has refocused attention on advocacy, and established a need to ensure that both patients' and carers' interests are served.

In many instances carers may take on the role of advocate, trying to ensure that patients are provided with the full range of services to which they are entitled. However, it may not always be possible for a carer to adequately or objectively assess patients' needs, nor may they know when standards are not being adequately met. Some local authorities are showing a lead in this field by allocating an independent advocate from a non-statutory agency (e.g. Immunity) to each client who has a care manager (Hammersmith and Fulham Borough Council, 1993), and greater use of such a system could be made in health-care provision.

POLICY AND RESEARCH ISSUES

Recent reforms of health and social services in the United Kingdom indicate a renewed emphasis on the community as the focus of continuing care. A plethora of White Papers, including *Working for Patients* (DoH, 1989b), *Caring for People* (DoH, 1989c), *Promoting Better Health* (DoH, 1987) and *Health of the Nation* (DoH, 1992), all make reference to the importance of community care.

Much of the research cited in this chapter emphasizes the need to enhance existing community nursing services by providing adequate training, supervision and support to individual nurses. This research also advocates the use of specialist nurses in HIV as sources of information and expertise, and as a resource for generic colleagues. The future of HIV community care will depend on a mixed economy of specialist and generic practitioners, working across professional boundaries and directly with patients and their informal carers.

At a time of great change in health care and of continuing developments in HIV treatment, there is a need to document and evaluate methods of service delivery. Although much can be done locally, particularly in terms of audit and outcome evaluation, larger-scale nursing research projects are required to ensure that progress is maintained. The majority of the research work discussed in this chapter has been commissioned by the Department of Health, and its importance to practice has been widely demonstrated.

Further consideration of research and development is made elsewhere in this book, but it needs to be stressed at this point that practitioners have a major responsibility in posing relevant research questions and formulating hypotheses for their academic colleagues to investigate. It is only with such collaboration that the service to people affected by HIV disease, whether carers, clients or patients, can be improved.

CONCLUSION

To those practitioners unfamiliar with HIV it may come as a relief to discover that many of the issues discussed in this chapter are not new and that solutions may be close at hand. Shared care, multidisciplinary discharge planning, clinical nurse specialists as resources and carer involvement have been integral parts of effective community care for many years. What is new, and even refreshing, is the vigour with which people affected by HIV have confronted professionals in the quest for high-quality care. The urgency of the epidemic has enabled research to take place into areas of nursing that have traditionally been regarded as low profile (e.g. district nursing, discharge planning).

Experience has shown that traditional primary care services are able to adapt to some of the more radical challenges posed by HIV, such as sexuality and drug misuse, but that specialist help is required for information, new skills training (e.g. for intravenous therapy) and support.

Evidence to date suggests that community nurses may be responding more effectively than their medical counterparts to the needs of people with HIV disease. Although some will derive satisfaction from such findings, there is a serious danger that comprehensive community care for this client group will become less rather than more effective should this state of affairs continue. On a rather more promising note, the experience gained by generic and specialist nurses in the field of HIV offers valuable lessons and provides many excellent examples to follow.

REFERENCES

Akinsanya, J.A. and Rouse, P. (1991) *Who Will Care? A Survey of the Knowledge and Attitudes of Hospital Nurses to People with HIV/AIDS.* Executive Summary. Health and Social Work Research Centre, Anglia Polytechnic, Chelmsford.

Armitage, S. and Jowett, S. (1988) *Hospital/Community Liaison Links in Nursing.* Unpublished Report, South Glamorgan Health Authority, Wales.

Bennett, C. and Pettigrew, A. (1991) *Pioneering Services for AIDS. The Response to HIV Infection in Four Health Authorities,* Centre for Corporate Strategy and Change, University of Warwick.

Bond, S. and Rhodes, T. (1990) HIV infection and community midwives: experience and practice. *Midwifery,* **6**, 33–40.

Bond, S., Rhodes, T., Philips, P. *et al.* (1991) Experience and preparation of community nursing staff for work associated with HIV infection and AIDS. *Social Science and Medicine,* **32**(1), 71–6.

Brocklehurst, N., Faugier, J., Butterworth, C.A. and Sloan, T. (1993) *Community Nursing Services for People Affected by HIV Disease.* 2nd Draft Report. University of Manchester.

Department of Health (1987) *Promoting Better Health.* Cm 249, HMSO, London.

Department of Health (1989a) *Discharge of Patients from Hospital.* HC (89) 5, HMSO, London.

Department of Health (1989b) *Working for Patients.* Cm 555, HMSO, London.

Department of Health (1989c) *Caring for People.* Cm 849, HMSO, London.

Department of Health (1992) *Health of the Nation: A Strategy for Health in England.* Cm 1986, HMSO, London.

Foy, C. and Gallagher, M. (1990) HIV and general practitioners: a national sample survey, in *AIDS Research: Handbook of Research and Development*, Department of Health, HMSO, London.

Hammersmith and Fulham Borough Council (1993) *Community Care Plan, 1993–1994*. Hammersmith and Fulham Social Services Department, London.

Haste, F.H. and Macdonald, L.D. (1992) The role of the specialist in community nursing: perceptions of specialist and district nurses. *International Journal of Nursing Studies*, 29(1), 37–47.

Hull–York Research Team (1993) *Social Care and HIV–AIDS*, Centre for Health Economics, Institute for Health Studies, HMSO, London.

Jowett, S, and Armitage, S. (1988) Hospital and community liaison links in nursing: the role of the liaison nurse. *Journal of Advanced Nursing*, 13, 579–87.

Quirk, J. and Reilly, G. (1993) Discharge planning and its effects on the setting for care for patients dying with AIDS. Poster presentation PO-B34-2312. IXth International Conference on AIDS, Berlin, 6–11 June, 1993.

Shailer, A., Butters, E. and George, R. (1993) *The UK Hospice Movement and HIV: A National Survey*. Poster presentation PO-B33-2297. IXth International Conference on AIDS. Berlin, 6–11 June, 1993.

Singleton, C. (1990) Primary health care liaison nursing. Forging vital links in care. *Nursing Standard*, 5(4), 25–7.

Smith, S., Parker, C., Ash, S. *et al.* (1993) *Development of a Model System for the Provision of HIV Health Care by Primary Care Physicians*. Poster presentation PO-B32-2263. IXth International Conference on AIDS. Berlin, 6–11 June 1993.

Tierney, A., Bond, S., Rhodes, T. and Philips, P. (1990) HIV infection, AIDS and community nursing staff in Scotland. *Health Bulletin*, 48(3), 114–23.

Waters, K. (1987) Outcomes of discharge from hospital for elderly people. *Journal of Advanced Nursing*, 12, 347–55.

Wolf, J. (1989) HIV and AIDS – who cares? *Journal of District Nursing*, June, 12–16.

Hospital services and HIV/AIDS

8

Margaret A. Worsley

INTRODUCTION

Since the first cases of AIDS were diagnosed in the USA in 1981, the exponential growth of this epidemic has created a public health crisis unparalleled in the latter half of this century (National League for Nursing, 1988). This has created a whole new set of challenges for all health workers, with nurses at the forefront. In 1988, Richard Wells identified the most important ones as:

- meaningful acute care in the hospital and the community;
- leaving control with or returning it to the patient;
- support for those close to the patient;
- confidentiality;
- patient advocacy.

It could be said that these challenges still exist for many nurses in practice today, along with the many ethical and moral dilemmas associated with the nursing management of people with AIDS (Mitchell and Smith, 1987; Goodman, 1990; Taravella, 1991). It is well established that patients with AIDS/HIV present with many problems that are best dealt with by staff other than doctors or nurses: indeed, most centres have adopted a multidisciplinary approach, and much more collaboration is evident than in the past, when staff and patients experienced secrecy-related problems which inhibited progress in nursing and medical practice (Bor *et al.*, 1989).

THE USE OF NURSING THEORY TO MEET PATIENTS' NEEDS

It is generally accepted that in any hospital setting the delivery of nursing care is based on an appropriate theoretical framework, although the profession is usually seen as practice orientated (Thibodeau, 1983). In 1952, Peplau described nursing as a significant therapeutic interpersonal process. She saw nursing as a human relationship between an individual who is sick, or in need of health services, and a nurse who is someone specially educated to recognize and to respond to the need for help (Peplau, 1952). Certain nursing writers argued that nursing models can form the starting point for the development of more rigorously tested theory (Chinn and Jacobs, 1983). Others have suggested that nurses can draw a distinction between nursing models which describe only aspects of people and nursing care, and ones that can predict the likely outcome of particular nursing strategies (Thibodeau, 1983). Thibodeau states that before one can talk about nursing models, one must understand the concept of paradigm, for it is from the paradigm for a given profession that the models for that profession are developed. The four components of the nursing paradigm have been described as:

- people
- environment
- health
- nursing.

It is accepted that other disciplines may address some of these topics, but all four must be included if a paradigm is to be considered a nursing paradigm (Thibodeau, 1983). The same writer states that there is no one dominant nursing paradigm that clearly guides the practice of the majority of nurses.

So what guides the practice of nursing for patients with AIDS? One can examine the theory of skill acquisition that is described by Dreyfus and Dreyfus (1980). This approach has been used by Benner (1984), who tried to analyse what makes an expert nurse. She gives a lucid description of nursing as practised by experts. Her work examines what nurses do in specific patient care situations and how beginners and experts do it differently. Benner identified seven domains of nursing practice which seem appropriate for the nursing of patients with HIV/AIDS. These are:

- the helping role;
- the teaching–coaching function;
- the diagnostic and patient-monitoring function;
- effective management of rapidly changing situations;
- administering and monitoring therapeutic interventions and regimens;
- monitoring and ensuring the quality of health-care practices;

- organizational and work-role competences.

Theory does guide nurses and enables them to ask the right questions, as is shown by the kind of transformation in practice. The field of oncology serves as a good model for this: in that field, nurses have moved slowly from a situation in which the cancer patient was totally dependent on the health team and the ambulatory care centre for treatment, monitoring and recovery, to one where patients have an active and independent role in their own care (Myers, 1988). Experience indicates that nursing theory offers explicit and formalized models, but clinical practice is always much more complex. I believe that, in the field of HIV/AIDS nursing, experience is essential in helping nurses develop intuitive skills, not merely as a result of the passage of time, but mainly because it allows nurses to refine preconceived notions and theory through encounters with actual aspects of patient care as described by Benner (1984). A practical example could be the use of nursing policies that are based on valid research but which may not be suitable for individual patients. The nurse should be able to prescribe the nursing care in collaboration with the patient and carers if appropriate, using the policy as a guide, as long as all the elements of safe practice are in place. The scope of professional practice does allow the nurse to be creative and flexible to meet the patient's needs to some extent (UKCC, 1993). Bergman (1990) and Salvage (1990) share the view that nurses should become more flexible and dispense with time-consuming rituals.

An American study describes some of the problems that really challenge nurses working in the field of HIV/AIDS. It was a qualitative study of the perspectives of doctors, nurses and social workers on terminally ill people with AIDS in their care. The methods used for this study were participant observation and focused interviews with professionals about dying patients whom they identified as being difficult to manage. It describes three patient types who were terminally ill, in relation to professional needs for cure or symptom amelioration, routine work and personal gratification. They found that the 'ideal' patients exceeded workers' expectations for response. The 'routine' patients conformed to normative expectations and presented conventional problems. The 'toxic' patients disrupted routines, had unattractive personal or disease characteristics, and questioned professional authority. This study may be flawed in the methodology but there are some similarities to the practice of HIV nursing in this country.

Personal experience indicates that the patient-led approach in the field of AIDS is still a shock to many nurses. Making it possible for the patient to be in control of the medical/nursing situation as described by Wells (1988) remains the exception rather than the rule. The unpopular or non-conforming patient is certainly not new to nurses, either in theory or in practice (Stockwell, 1972). Providing effective, compassionate and high-quality nursing care which is patient centred and based on valid research remains paramount. How this is delivered in hospital has to be fairly individual in nature. There are some excellent examples in the literature where patients' records and their experiences in hospital have been used to audit and ultimately improve the quality of care (Cleary *et al.*, 1992; Butters *et al.*, 1993; Hutchinson, 1991).

PATIENT EDUCATION

There is a need to research the very particular needs of people who have to go through repeated hospital admissions as a result of HIV disease. Individuals are often ill prepared for the effects of the disease process on their lives, hence the importance of establishing what type of support and information they require.

Patient education constitutes a vital part of medical and nursing care: research on its effectiveness has by now produced many reviews which, almost without exception, emphasize its role as an effective intervention (Redman, 1993). As more and more patients with HIV disease become active in making decisions about their treatment, they need appropriate education (Redman, 1993). In the field of oncology, some authors have developed a test to assess knowledge about treatment options (Ward and Griffin, 1990). Programmes to educate siblings about cancer and its treatment could be used as a model for patients with HIV-related disease. A study carried out in San Francisco by Lovejoy and Moran (1988) revealed that 90% of patients reported a need for further information about various parts of their care. Quality of life indicators have not been reported conclusively in the field of HIV, although some work by a team in California can be used as an example of an effective education programme for the prevention of infection (Karl and Eck, 1990). A survey of cancer rehabilitation programmes found patient education to be the most common feature among all the institutions involved in the study (Harvey *et al.*, 1981). There are excellent examples of model programmes that have been developed to help families care for cancer patients at home or to help patients cope with the disease (Redman and Braun, 1991). These programmes could be transferred effectively to patient education and HIV disease. It is widely accepted in the literature (Luker and Caress, 1989) that appropriate patient education is an important nursing function and an integral part of the professional scope of practice (UKCC, 1993).

ACCESSING FUNDING TO DEVELOP SERVICES

Service development in the future will depend on the quality of information provided for the purchaser of the service. In terms of the nursing service in the hospital situation, consideration will have to be given to a continuous quality improvement programme (Rosso, 1984) which clearly develops outcome indicators in collaboration with the users of the service. Such a programme should provide a high-quality service and a system for consistent good-quality data which can be used by purchasers, and indeed client groups, to differentiate between providers. Bringing the method of funding for HIV/AIDS into line with the mainstream purchaser–provider relationship will have important benefits, and units should seize this opportunity to compete in the market.

One publication (McCarthy and Layzell, 1993) suggests that maintaining the quality of the existing services while enabling trusts with low prevalence to develop their own means that HIV and AIDS coordinators will in effect become purchasing authorities. These people could then contract for services on behalf of the local population. This is a very subjective opinion, and one could argue that close collaboration between purchaser and provider would maximize health gain without the need for an individual post. Many hospital units have encouraged self-referral, and sought to make best use of the service by ensuring confidentiality.

The debate about the use of centralized services in big hospitals is still going on: these clearly provide benefits in the quality of service, but conversely local services remain underdeveloped, which ultimately causes problems for HIV-infected patients who find it difficult to travel for treatment, such as people with young families and economic problems. Many hospitals in the USA have examined the value of dedicated units, i.e. the physical designation of a nursing unit for the care of people with AIDS and HIV disease, and the use of a dedicated team of staff comprising all disciplines (Pellegrino and Spicehandler, 1988; McCaffrey, 1987). According to one team (Rothman and Tynan, 1990), there are many advantages to designated HIV/AIDS units. They claim that such units do not seem to stigmatize the patients or reduce the quality of care, while still allowing the patient a real choice. Recruitment of staff does not seem to be a problem and student nurses and doctors gain invaluable clinical experience. On the other hand, in areas of low prevalence patients generally do not want to be labelled by attending a special unit.

HIV/AIDS HOSPITAL CARE AND CLINICAL AUDIT

Measuring the quality of life of people with AIDS is becoming increasingly important as the treatment of opportunistic infections improves and people are living longer (Fanning and Emmott, 1993). The focus has now moved from measuring the effects of HIV infection and treatments solely in symptom management terms to assessing the impact of the illness and treatment interventions on the person's social, psychological and economic well-being. Current quality of life indicators are not significantly sensitive to the very complex issues affecting people with AIDS and HIV disease. However, despite the absence of well-researched quality of life indicators, nursing staff in hospital settings can still examine quality measurements in clinical practice. There are examples of standard setting and care planning which could be used as a good starting point (Barry, 1988; Johns, 1989). Funding in this country will only be allocated for projects that are multidisciplinary in nature and can be described as clinical audit. The subject of audit is now orthodox, and many of the Royal Colleges stipulate that training posts for junior staff will only be recognized if there is an active audit programme within each unit (Crombie *et al.*, 1993). Although all practitioners are now officially encouraged to audit their practice, it would be unfortunate if staff only did it for this reason. Purchasing authorities are already requesting the results of clinical audits. The discerning staff in purchasing teams will be examining methods associated with clinical audit as a means to improve the service. Systems of clinical audit are not well established yet, but in the meantime nursing staff in hospitals should already be leading the way in producing protocols for nursing practice, formulated by all grades of staff and including patient representatives. These protocols should be based on up-to-date nursing research and contain achievable safe standards before being implemented in clinical areas. Finally, their efficacy should be measured by means of an appropriate audit tool.

One of the key questions in any quality assurance system is who is going to set the standard and then measure the outcome. There appears to be no conflict about the formulation of standards, the consensus being that clinical nurses should decide and lead their individual practice (UKCC, 1993). However, personal experience indicates that many nurses are very uneasy about introducing a system of peer review, which can be applied either to an individual or a team. Although both approaches form elements of quality control, the group approach can quite clearly be seen to be part of quality assurance, whereas the individual one may appear as a management process, forming part of an appraisal or a system of individual performance review. Mullins *et al.* (1979) list the purposes of peer review as being:

- to establish an objective means for providing evaluation feedback to individual nurses;
- to recognize the individual nurse who has outstanding nursing skills and performs at a high level of clinical practice;
- to identify individual areas of the nurse's practice that need further development;
- to analyse the consistency of the individual nurse's practice compared to accepted professional standards.

The criteria described could be used effectively in the field of HIV/AIDS nursing in hospital. Has the time come for nurses in HIV/AIDS units to join forces and set up a formal system of peer review?

Some would argue that it is impossible to compare like with like, but surely elements of research-based clinical nursing practice could be measured, and the outcomes used on a national basis to improve HIV/AIDS nursing practice (Bennett, 1987; Smeed, 1990; Wilmsmeyer, 1990; Waites and Mello, 1991; Arkell, 1993).

EDUCATION, NURSES AND HOSPITAL CARE

Several studies have highlighted the inadequacy of knowledge among nurses and other health-care workers (Morgan and Treadway, 1989; Klimes *et al.*, 1989; Henry *et al.*, 1990; Carreta *et al.*, 1990; Sullivan *et al.*, 1991; Cole and Slocumb, 1993; Wissen and Siebers, 1993; Plant and Foster, 1993).

Gallop *et al.* (1992) maintain that nurses' fear of contagion remains quite high despite increased levels of knowledge. The findings in this study suggest that familiarity with the illness and knowledge of universal infection control precautions do not seem to be effective in reducing fear of contagion. According to Flaskerud (1989), many education programmes are ineffective for individuals with negative attitudes towards AIDS patients. Exercises for changing attitudes, including discussion groups, attitude examination exercises and role modelling, have been shown to have some effect. The work completed by Cole and Slocumb (1993) highlights the problems that nurses appear to have when they decide how the patient became HIV positive.

According to other workers, because AIDS is associated with a stigma that already exists in people, the disease provokes reactions similar to those against gay men, drug users, racial minorities or outsiders in general (Herek and Glunt, 1988). However, this did not feature in the work by Wissen and Siebers (1993) in New Zealand, which suggests that further work is needed to analyse attitudes.

Research in the UK (Akinsanya and Rouse, 1992) demonstrated that a great number of nurses were very ill informed about AIDS. Once again, personal experience shows that, in areas of low prevalence of the disease, many staff have problems when faced with patients in a clinical situation. One of the major gaps still appears to be knowledge and skills associated with injecting drug users. Nurses appear ready to accept gay men as patients but remain wary of drug users (Brettle, 1990; Lert and Marne, 1992), and yet, in most parts of the country nurses have easy access to further specialized education.

MANAGING CHANGE

A team of American nurses stated: 'We must move the patient to the top of the chart; once the patient is valued, the nurse who delivers care to the patient will be valued as well'. These nurses set out to search for excellence, pointing out that nurses need to know they have made a difference, and that the nurse–physician relationship should be supportive, constructive and collegial (American Journal of Nursing, 1987).

Nurses caring for people with HIV/AIDS need to work in collaboration with the multidisciplinary team and the patients in order to continue to develop and make progress. Some alterations will have to be made in order to take into account the major changes in health-care provision. Management of change is well documented in the literature (Archer et al., 1984). Most of us dislike changes in routine, and will only adopt a favourable attitude to them if there is some probable gain to be achieved. Many uncertainties surrounding change are based on inadequate information. There are many changes affecting nurses: those working with HIV/AIDS patients are uncertain about the available funding in the future (McCarthy and Layzell, 1993).

The recently introduced changes in community care have made effective discharge planning a vital component of nursing care from the time of admission to the hospital. Nursing is also increasingly affected by patient-focused initiatives and their impact on the role of the generic nurse. The patient-focused approach is built on the concept of decentralization of the delivery of care. The overall management of care should lie with the team who delivers it, in partnership with the patient. Such care can be adapted to the hospital or the community. In hospitals, this might mean the decentralization of equipment in order to bring services and activities closer to the patient, leading to the development of a care delivery system that brings together all staff concerned.

In theory, some elements of patient-focused care already exist in the field of HIV/AIDS nursing. The recent guidance from the Department of Health points the way clearly for nurses in the foreseeable future (NHSME, 1993a). The targets set out in *A Vision for the Future* are already being examined in most provider units. Many can be used by clinical nurses to help them access resources for enhancing their nursing practice, for example research-based practice and clinical supervision (Butterworth and Faugier, 1992).

It is clear that the NHS reforms have increased the pressure to find outcome measures for nursing that will enable purchasers and providers to specify relationships between ward resources, the organization of nursing care and quality. In the absence of dependable outcome measures for nursing people with HIV/AIDS, we should concentrate on the reliable research to date, and work with academic departments to develop ways of continuing meaningful research in HIV/AIDS nursing practice.

REFERENCES

Akinsanya, J. and Rouse, P. (1992) Who will care? A survey of the knowledge and attitudes of hospital nurses to people with AIDS. *Journal of Advanced Nursing*, **17**, 464–71.

American Journal of Nursing (1987) Transcript from Conference. Nurses for the future searching for excellence. *American Journal of Nursing*, December, 1638–48.

Archer, S.E., Kelly, C.D. and Bisch, S.A. (1984) *Implementing Change in Communities. A Collaborative Process*, CV Mosby, St Louis.

Arkell, S. (1993) Health care delivery for people with HIV infection and AIDS. *British Journal of Nursing*, **2**(21), 1065–9.

Audit Commission (1991) *The Virtue of Patients: Making Best Use of Ward Nursing Resources*, HMSO, London.

Barry, A. (1988) AIDS. A nursing care plan. *Infection Control Canada*, March–April, 10–14.

Benner, P. (1984) *From Novice to Expert*, Addison-Wesley, Menlo Park, California.

Bennett, J.O. (1987) Nurses talk about the challenge of AIDS. *American Journal of Nursing*, September, 1150–5.

Bergman, R. (1990) Thoughts on the future of nursing. *Journal of Advanced Nursing*, **15**, 865–6.

Bor, R., Miller, R. and Salt, H. (1989) Secrecy-related problems in AIDS management. *Journal of the Royal College of Physicians of London*, **23**(4), 264–7.

Brettle, R.P. (1990) Hospital health care for HIV infection with particular reference to injecting drug users. *AIDS Care*, **2**(2), 171–81.

Butters, E., Higginson, I., George, R. and McCarthy, M. (1993) Palliative care for people with HIV/AIDS: views of patients, carers and providers. *AIDS Care*, **5**(1), 105–16.

Butterworth, T. and Faugier, J. (1992) *Clinical Supervision*, Chapman & Hall, London.

Carreta, R.A., Mangione, T.W., Marson, P.F. and Darmono, S.S. (1990) AIDS education practices among Massachusetts physicians. *Journal of Community Health*, **15**(3), 147–62.

Chinn, P. and Jacobs, M. (1983) *Theory and Nursing – a Systematic Approach*, CV Mosby, St Louis.

Cleary, P.D., Fahs, M.C., McMullen, W.G. *et al.* (1992) Using patient reports to assess hospital treatment of persons with AIDS: a pilot study. *AIDS Care*, **4**(3), 325–32.

Cole, F.L. and Slocumb, E.M. (1993) Nurses' attitudes toward patients with AIDS. *Journal of Advanced Nursing*, **18**, 1112–17.

Crombie, I.K., Davis, H.T.O., Abraham, S.C.S. and Florey, C. duV. (1993) *The Audit Handbook*, Wiley, Chichester.

Dreyfus, S.E. and Dreyfus, H.L. (1980) *A Five Stage Model of the Mental Activities Involved in Directed Skill Acquisition*, USAF, University of California.

Fanning, M.A. and Emmott, S. (1993) Evaluation of a quality of life instrument for HIV/AIDS. *AIDS Patient Care*, **7**(3), 161–2.

Flaskerud, J.H. (1989) *AIDS/HIV Infection*, WB Saunders, London.

Gallop, R.M., Lancee, W.J., Taerk, G. *et al.* (1992) Fear of contagion and AIDS: nurses' perception of risk. *AIDS Care*, **4**(1), 103–9.

Goodman, H.G.(1990) Death work: Staff perspectives on the care of terminally ill patients in an acute care hospital. *Dissertation Abstracts International A*, **51**(3), 1002.

Harvey, R.F., Jellinek, H.M. and Habeck, R.V. (1981) Cancer rehabilitation. An analysis of 36 program approaches. *JAMA*, **247**, 2127–31.

Henry, K., Campbell, S. and Willenbring, K. (1990) A cross-sectional analysis of variables impacting on AIDS related knowledge, attitudes, and behaviors among employees of a Minnesota teaching hospital. *AIDS Education Preview*, **2**(1), 36–47.

Herek, G.M. and Glunt, E.K. (1988) An epidemic of stigma: public reactions to AIDS. *American Psychologist*, **43**, 886–91.

HMSO (1993) *The Health and Social Care of People with HIV Infection and AIDS*, HMSO, London.

Hutchison, M. (1991) 'I need to know that I have a choice'. *AIDS Patient Care*, **5**(1), 17–25.

Johns, C. (1989) Setting standards for performance review. *Surgical Nurse*, July, 528.

Karl, S.B. and Eck, E.K. (1990) Living healthy with HIV. A patient education program whose time has come. *Group Practice Journal*, **39**(1), 31–5.

Klimes, I., Catalan, J., Bond, A. and Day, A. (1989) Knowledge and attitudes of health care staff about HIV infection in a health district with low HIV prevalence. *AIDS Care*, **1**(3), 313–18.

Lert, F. and Marne, M.J. (1992) Hospital care for drug users with AIDS or HIV infection in France. *AIDS Care*, **4**(3), 333–8.

Lovejoy, N, and Moran, T. (1988) Informational needs and behaviors of men with AIDS or ARC. *Oncology Nursing Forum*, **15**(2) (suppl), 104.

Luker, K. and Caress, A.L. (1989) Rethinking patient education. *Journal of Advanced Nursing*, **14**, 711–18.

Mangan, P. (1993) A dream ticket? *Nursing Times*, **89**(29), 27–8.

McCaffrey, E. (1987) Setting up an AIDS unit. *AIDS Patient Care*, **1**(1), 6–8.

McCarthy, M. and Layzell, S. (1993) Funding policies for HIV and AIDS: time for change. *British Medical Journal*, **307**, 367–71.

Mitchell, C. and Smith, L. (1987) If it's AIDS, please don't tell. *American Journal of Nursing*, July, 911–15.

Morgan, K.J. and Treadway, J. (1989) Surveying nursing staff's attitudes about AIDS. *AIDS Patient Care*, **3**(5), 34–8.

Mullins, A.C., Colavecchio, R.E. and Tescher, B.E. (1979) Peer review: a model for professional accountability. *Journal of Nursing Administration*, December, 25–30.

Myers, P.A. (1988) Patient teaching models for outpatient self-management of interferon. *Oncology Nursing Forum*, **15**(2), (suppl), 131.

National League for Nursing (1988) *AIDS Guidelines for Schools of Nursing*, National League for Nursing, New York.

NHSME (1993a) *A Vision for the Future*, HMSO, London.

NHSME (1993b) *Report of the Task Force on the Strategy for Research in Nursing, Midwifery and Health Visiting*, HMSO, London.

Pellegrino, V. and Spicehandler, D. (1988) Dedicated AIDS units: pros and cons. *AIDS Patient Care*, **2**(2), 8–11.

Peplau, H.E. (1952) *Interpersonal Relations in Nursing*, GP Putnam's Sons, New York.

Plant, M. and Foster, J. (1993) AIDS related experience, knowledge, attitudes and beliefs among nurses in an area with a high rate of HIV infection. *Journal of Advanced Nursing*, **18**, 80–8.

Redman, B.K. (1993) Patient education at 25 years: where we have been and where we are going. *Journal of Advanced Nursing*, **18**, 725–30.

Redman, B.K. and Braun, R. (1991) Courses in patient education in master's programs in nursing. *Journal of Nursing Education*, **30**(1), 42–3.

Rosso, M.S. (1984) Knowledge of practice: the state of clinical research, in *Measuring the Quality of Care*, (eds L.D. Willis and M.E. Linwood), Churchill Livingstone, Edinburgh, pp. 43–65.

Rothman, D.J. and Tynan, E.A. (1990) Special report: advantages and disadvantages of special hospitals for patients with HIV infection. A report by the New York City Task Force on single-disease hospitals. *New England Journal of Medicine*, **323**, 764–8.

Rowden, R. (1993) Breaking the mould. *Nursing Times*, **89**(29), 29–30.

Salvage, J. (1990) Nurses: the point of no return. *British Medical Journal*, **300**, 1478.

Smeed, C. (1990) Use of a midline catheter in PWAs. *AIDS Patient Care*, **4**(3), 34–7.

Stockwell, F. (1972) *The Unpopular Patient*, RCN, London.

Sullivan, C., Campbell, S. and Henry, K. (1991) Assimilation of recent knowledge about HIV/AIDS by physicians and nurses at a US ID teaching hospital: a comparative analysis. International Conference on AIDS, 16–21 June.

Taravella, S. (1991) AIDS care programs struggle as grant funding runs out. *Models of Healthcare*, **21**(7), 26–7.

Thibodeau, J.A. (1983) *Nursing Models: Analysis and Evaluation*, Wadsworth, California.

UKCC (1993) *Scope of Professional Practice*, UKCC, London.

Waites, L. and Mello, L. Long-term parenteral nutrition support in a 30 year old man. *AIDS Patient Care*, **5**(2), 60–1.

Ward, S. and Griffin, J. (1990) Developing a test of knowledge of surgical options for breast cancer. *Cancer Nurse*, **13**, 191–6.

Wells, R. (1988) Are nurses ready to meet the challenge? *Senior Nurse*, **8**, 6–7.

Wilmsmeyer, D. (1990) Nursing management of the AIDS patient. *AIDS Patient Care*, **4**(3), 22–5.

Wissen, K.A. and Siebers, R.W.L. (1993) Nurses' attitudes and concerns pertaining to HIV and AIDS. *Journal of Advanced Nursing*, **18**, 912–17.

Models of care 9

Part a: Inpatient care

Carol Smith

INTRODUCTION

'The greatest misery of sickness is solitude; when the infectiousness of the disease deters them who should assist from coming' (John Donne, 1627).

John Donne's observation was made in 1627, in reference to syphilis; yet it appears pertinent to health service reaction to the AIDS pandemic three centuries later. Hospitals were the first institutions to encounter AIDS, and the early response to those affected by a new and poorly understood disease was variable. Some rose to the challenge by developing services in response to need, while others tried to avoid or ignore the problem. When recording of UK statistics commenced in 1984, HIV disease was thought to exclusively affect homosexual men. Evidence of discrimination and intolerance by health-care workers in response to perceived threats is illustrated by attempts to institute widespread HIV testing of these patients. The picture of those infected with HIV has changed, and in the 12-month period to January 1994, heterosexual men and women accounted for 38% of HIV infections reported (PHLS, 1994).

In Britain, inpatient HIV care models have developed in accordance with geographical area, the amount of HIV patient activity and hospital resources. Increasing admissions of patients with HIV disease in the 1980s led to the creation of dedicated units, largely in London, Edinburgh and Glasgow.

Patients travelled to metropolitan areas rather than utilize local services because of a perception that greater experience in treating HIV disease would equal better treatment, and assumptions that geographical distance would mean that anonymity would be preserved more easily – critical from the patient's viewpoint, given the stigma associated with HIV/AIDS. However, increasing care distribution throughout the UK has led to acute services such as infectious disease units, haematology units, departments of genitourinary medicine, gastroenterology and respiratory services integrating HIV services in district general/local hospitals where dedicated units are not practicable. The debate on whether 'specialist dedicated' or 'generalist non-dedicated' units should provide HIV services remains a controversial one: Table 9.1 compares the perceived benefits and disadvantages of the two approaches.

Table 9.1 The benefits and disadvantages of dedicated versus general units

Dedicated units – benefits

- Development of specialized, focused service, expertise in field
- Nurses highly motivated to work with people affected by HIV/AIDS
- Confidentiality generally easier to maintain

Disadvantages

- Elitism
- Less opportunity for skill sharing with other departments
- Decreased anonymity – unit publicly identified as 'AIDS unit', even when euphemisms are employed such as communicable diseases ward
- Risks ghettoizing – general units opting out of AIDS care, reinforces mystique, and may help perpetuate myths
- Staff burnout

General wards – benefits

- Anonymity – more difficult to identify HIV patients
- Skill sharing
- Inevitability, as more people affected and survival rates increase, dedicated units will become impractical

- With hands-on experience, likely that increased confidence will reduce anxiety and fear around nursing people with HIV
- Possible 'normalizing' of HIV

Disadvantages

- Patient isolation – no identification with, and support from other patients affected
- As staff have not chosen to work in the field, attitudes less predictable
- Staff may hold religious or moral viewpoints which negatively influence attitudes to patients
- Difficult for staff to remain clinically up to date if they only rarely nurse patients with HIV
- Confidentiality more difficult to maintain because of attendant fears/perception of infection risk by staff and the 'need to know' within multidisciplinary setting
- Inappropriate precautions taken as a response to fear of contagion – (e.g. a health-care assistant refusing to help an AIDS patient who had fallen out of bed before drawing on two pairs of gloves)

The management and working practices of dedicated units and infection control issues are well documented elsewhere in this book. This chapter will therefore focus on the management of HIV services in non-dedicated units and consider key factors in providing inpatient care.

HOSPITAL HIV MANAGEMENT STRATEGIES

In line with Department of Health policy, hospitals are attempting to develop services which meet the needs of identified client groups while acknowledging the need to provide the highest-quality service to their entire catchment population. HIV-related services aim to develop according to an explicit strategy, with an overall aim of enabling staff to provide effective treatment, care and prevention services as perceived by both the providers and the users. However, there are difficulties in reconciling national and local health targets as Government priorities (to prevent the wider spread of HIV into the majority heterosexual population) compete with regional priorities, such as direct health-care service provision for affected groups.

ORGANIZING INPATIENT CARE

HIV is a useful barometer of health service responses to the needs of traditionally disadvantaged groups in that it has challenged the NHS to create new and dynamic solutions to complex issues. Given the range of needs of people living with HIV/AIDS and the wide spectrum of services provided by different professional groups, there is clearly a need for coordination of hospital services in the light of knowledge about the resident population. One model which has evolved in the development of HIV inpatient services is the multidisciplinary coordinating committee. This forum recognizes that there are ethical, professional and employment concerns to be addressed in managing HIV-related issues which require interdepartmental collaboration. Such committees may have representatives from the occupational health, genitourinary medicine, infection control, microbiology, medical and surgical departments to develop shared care policies and joint protocols for the management of patients with HIV disease. Nurses are a vital part of this structure, because traditionally they act as the interface between the patient and other professionals, and act as the coordinators of care; a useful example is the management of HIV-positive pregnant women to facilitate access to HIV services and streamline the number of hospital visits women and their families make, and developing facilities for a sick parent and child to be nursed in the same department.

MEETING DIVERSE PATIENT NEEDS

Decisions about the most appropriate ways of organizing hospital services have generally been based on local HIV prevalence and projected patient numbers. Typically, inpatient care for those with HIV infection or AIDS is integrated with other acute services provided on general wards within district general hospitals. Patients are admitted to one of the medical wards, and inpatient care is provided by specialist teams to cover the spectrum of HIV disease. For example, HIV care might be jointly managed by the genitourinary medicine and thoracic teams, ensuring continuity between inpatient and outpatient services; following discharge, care would be continued by the genitourinary physicians, along with the appropriate community services.

Certain epidemiological patterns are emerging, and although the heterosexual spread of HIV is increasing steadily the epidemic has concentrated among men who have sex with men, injecting drug users and attenders of genitourinary clinics (PHLS, 1991). There is a wide regional variation in the incidence of HIV: London is disproportionately affected in terms of prevalence among gay men, and much of the pioneering work of specialist units was in partnership with this group. Recent epidemiological data have assisted in identifying other groups whose needs are not currently met, such as women, children and minority ethnic groups.

Although HIV services have developed in conjunction with, and will need to continue to be targeted towards, gay men, consideration needs to be given to the specific needs of heterosexual women, men and their families in the development of inpatient services.

SERVICES FOR WOMEN

The clinical presentation of HIV disease appears similar in both women and men. However, it is clear that women have other issues that need consideration on the ward, such as:

- women being traditionally regarded as 'carers' who now need care themselves;
- child care and the future of orphans;
  confidentiality for themselves and their families;
  future social/sexual acceptability;
- contraceptive options, fertility, pregnancy and breastfeeding.

These concerns may be in addition to typical symptomatology – weight loss, diarrhoea, nutritional needs, oral infections, skin lesions, cerebral symptoms and gynaecological conditions. There are very few straightforward answers to any of these issues, but resources such as helplines, voluntary agencies and support groups are all valuable. Self-help groups may be particularly useful in terms of advocacy and support. In terms of service development, close alliances with gynaecology and family planning services are essential. There are also practical ward considerations, such as encouraging **all** women patients to handle and dispose of their own sanitary protection.

BLACK AND MINORITY ETHNIC PEOPLE

There is no evidence whatsoever to indicate that HIV susceptibility has a racial basis. However, there is substantial evidence to suggest that AIDS follows social and economic lines of frailty. The overrepresentation of minority ethnic people in cases of AIDS merits concerted action to develop appropriate services, but there are difficulties in targeting AIDS services without simultaneously stigmatizing an already marginal group.

Particular problems presenting themselves in the continuing care of black and ethnic minority patients are poor housing, social support networks and communication difficulties due to language and cultural differences. Patients may require intensive counselling and education with regard to the disease, as HIV may not be the most urgent priority in their lives. Access to interpreting services, the provision of information in minority languages which is acceptable to the cultural and religious beliefs of black and ethnic minority people, and HIV/AIDS palliative care which takes into account their beliefs, customs and values, are all areas in which nurses are well placed to develop and expand services.

STAFF TRAINING

The compassion which is often extended to those who are likely to die may be denied to people with AIDS. Studies looking at lay people's and health workers' perceptions of different illnesses found that AIDS patients were the most negatively evaluated and the most rejected. Rattigan (1991) nicely illustrates this point with his story of how, as a psychotherapist new to a unit caring for HIV-positive patients, he was welcomed by the staff as the ideal medium for getting affected patients to face up to their 'wickedness'.

The need for ongoing in-service education is widely acknowledged and has been exhaustively documented. In a recent audit compiled by the author, nurses reported an active interest in the subject and a general willingness to attend for education and training. However, on analysis nurses reported difficulties in attending because they risked leaving the wards short-staffed, and a considerable number reported attending in their own time. These findings underline the need for adequate resources to ensure that staff cover is available to release staff for appropriate training.

STAFF SUPPORT

People affected by HIV infection are part of a complex set of cultural, emotional and social dynamics, the diversity of which may be overwhelming for the health-care worker. Ethical concerns such as HIV testing and confidentiality within the ward setting have consistently been identified as difficult areas. However, caring for the patient with HIV disease does not usually require that the nurse learn new skills. Support to boost confidence, and the provision of a forum in which staff may address individual concerns and obtain accurate, up-to-date information on HIV-related issues, are the most important factors.

HIV TESTING

When there is clinical suspicion of HIV infection confirmatory tests will be requested. It is standard practice to undertake pretest counselling where the medical, social employment and insurance implications of a positive HIV antibody test are explained. In a number of hospitals this is undertaken by health advisers or clinical nurse specialists, who provide an 'on-call' service to wards to ensure that appropriate information is given, and who may provide psychological support after a positive diagnosis. Emphasis should be placed on **informed** consent, as compulsory testing in any context is unethical, ineffective, unnecessarily intrusive, discriminatory and counterproductive. Effective teamwork is essential to this complex process, for example in supporting patients and providing practical advice if they are considering when and how to tell relatives of a positive result.

CONFIDENTIALITY

Confidentiality is crucial for all patients regardless of their illness, and actively seeking permission to share information is an integral part of involving the patient in decision making. As all staff should be aware of what constitutes good practice in relation to infection control, there should be no reason to disclose antibody status to ensure that staff are 'protected' – the usual argument put forward for disclosure of HIV status. The consequences of failure to maintain confidentiality are well documented: physical attacks, unwelcome media attention and irrevocable damage to relationships. Protecting patient privacy is essential to preserving nurse–patient relationships. Patients are unlikely to access services if they doubt the standards of confidentiality on the ward.

CONCLUSION

Aligning the ideals of autonomy and quality of inpatient care with such a diversity of patient needs seems something of a daunting task, requiring a broad range of skills within the ward team. However, there is a wealth of evidence to suggest that nurses already exercise innovation and flexibility in their nursing practice: for example, some nurses have undertaken complementary therapy training courses in massage and aromatherapy in their own time. HIV disease presents a range of clinical symptoms which require an equally broad repertoire of interventions. The course of an individual's disease may be erratic, and AIDS patients live with constant uncertainty. Until vaccines appear, nursing and medical care is the most valuable tool available to keep well those that are affected and enable patients to make informed decisions about their lives.

REFERENCES

Donne, J. (1627) *Devotions Upon Emergent Occasions*.
Public Health Laboratory Service (1991) *Quarterly AIDS and HIV Figures*. News Release, June.
Public Health Laboratory Service (1994) *Quarterly AIDS and HIV Figures*. News Release, January.
Rattigan, B. (1991) On not traumatising th traumatised: the contribution of psychodynamic psychotherapy to work with people with HIV and AIDS. *British Journal of Psychotherapy*, **8**(1), 40–7.

Part b: Day and respite care

Sarah Holmes-Smith

INTRODUCTION

The day care service at London Lighthouse was developed to meet the needs of people living with HIV-related psychological and/or neurological problems, who are vulnerable at home and require nursing care and support throughout the day. The service opened in January 1991 in response to an identified gap in the balance of services offered by London Lighthouse and other statutory and voluntary organizations. As such, the service is seen as complementing existing service provision.

LONDON LIGHTHOUSE

London Lighthouse, Britain's first major residential and support centre for men and women affected by HIV and AIDS, opened in November 1988. The project is based in a specially designed building off Ladbroke Grove in west London. Staff are committed to providing the best possible care, support and facilities so that people affected by HIV can live their lives to the full.

The project was set up in 1986 by a group of people who were living with HIV and AIDS, or who knew people who were. They saw the need for a centre where such people could be supported to live well, have control over their lives, and make key decisions about the organization and its quality and range of services. People affected by HIV and AIDS are involved throughout the organization. London Lighthouse also supports the partners, friends and families of people affected by HIV and AIDS.

PROJECT PHILOSOPHY

There are three main commitments which form the basis of London Lighthouse's operational philosophy:

- to build into all our activities time and space for the giving and receiving of care and attention between individuals and groups;
- to work to change deep-rooted attitudes which deny that death and dying are central to life and living;
- to challenge prejudice and oppression.

In addition to the day care service London Lighthouse provides a range of support services, including residential care, home support, counselling, support groups, complementary and creative therapies, housing and welfare services, and drop-in facilities. These services aim to assist people with HIV to make and sustain immunosupportive changes in their lives.

BALANCING CARE

When developing the day-care service it was necessary to consider various factors that needed balancing when providing care. This is still being done in response to constant changes in legislation, health and social services, and the epidemiology of HIV. There is a question of balance between:

- hospital and home;
- meeting the individual's physical, mental, emotional and spiritual needs;
- structure and unstructure;
- throughput, quality and outcome;
- being user led and being purchaser led.

WHO THE SERVICE IS FOR

Historically, the majority of health-care service provision for people with HIV-related disease was carried out by hospital-based units (Adler, 1987), and resources have been concentrated on dealing with the physical aspects of the disease and its 'outpatient' treatment. There has now developed a range of self-help drop-in centres, counselling services and home care/support teams. However, this still left a gap in services for people who are vulnerable at home and need nursing care and support throughout the day. The day-care service therefore aims to enable people with HIV infection to achieve a high level of independent living with an improved quality of life while remaining in the community.

The service uses five criteria for admission, assessment and care programme formation:

- rehabilitation – for people who have had a period of illness and need some help to re-establish their routine;
- respite – for people who are living alone or with a carer and who need a break from coping with the burden of this;
- crisis – for people who are going through extremely difficult or traumatic circumstances of a temporary nature;
- psychological adjustment – for example depression and anxiety states, usually preceded by a loss of some kind;
- ongoing support – for people with a marked need for ongoing support, probably because of impairments caused by HIV-related central nervous system disease.

MODEL OF CARE

When developing a model of care for the service the team felt it was important that the model should be flexible enough to meet the needs of people with very different emotional and physical problems, as each person's experience of HIV disease is unique. The model also needed to incorporate the needs of service users who were moving towards stability or health, and those whose condition was deteriorating and who were in the process of dying. The model was initially developed by Ryan in 1991, when the service first opened, and is being updated as the service becomes more established.

The therapeutic interventions of the team vary according to the needs of the individual, in some cases supporting a move towards independence, in others helping people to accept the resources and support they will need to die peacefully, with dignity and with as much control as they would like. Care is directed at the whole person: their physical, mental, emotional and spiritual needs since although for some the move towards physical health may no longer be possible, it may be possible to provide emotional and spiritual healing and move towards mental health.

The model of care aims to:

- make full use of the team's multidisciplinary skills;
- maintain the rights and obligations of the individual service users and team members;
- acknowledge the individuality of people using the service;
- enable the self-identification of needs;

- encourage negotiations between service users and key workers in formulating and evaluating care programmes;
- maintain commitment to challenging the disempowering effects of prejudice and oppression.

STRUCTURE OF SERVICE

As London Lighthouse is care and support based, the service is nursing led and draws upon the established expertise of nursing in providing a holistic approach to individualized care. Duplication of services is avoided, which is particularly important in the current changing financial climate. With the introduction of care in the community legislation and the contract culture, even greater effort is required to ensure effective liaison and coordination between all service providers involved with each person using the day care service.

The Group Head, who is psychiatric- and general nurse-trained, has responsibility for the day-to-day management of the service. The staff team consists of trained nurses, an occupational therapist, an administrator and trained volunteers. Sessional staff include a medical officer, and complementary therapists such as masseurs, an acupuncturist, an aromatherapist, a reflexologist and a relaxation and stress therapist. All full-time staff have additional training or are supervised in working with people with mental health problems.

Referrals are accepted from any agencies or individuals as long as they have the person's permission. Due to limited resources and changes in funding arrangements, the service is increasingly having to accept only those people referred from an authority with which London Lighthouse has a contractual agreement.

The services on offer in the day care unit include the opportunity for one-to-one support sessions, often in the morning and sometimes including the person's carer. Complementary therapy sessions occur throughout the day, and individual and group occupational therapy sessions – for example in stress and anxiety management, and creative and social therapies – take place in the afternoons. Dietary advice and a free nutritious meal is available. There is a women-only day, with child-care provision. Some transport is provided through volunteer drivers and the use of taxis. At the present time there are places for 10 people a day and the service usually carries an active caseload of 48 people, with an overall occupancy rate of 93%.

A range of people use the service in terms of background, culture, interests and needs, so there is a constant requirement to accommodate the different tastes, value systems and support required. Staff work to reduce any tension that may arise to ensure that individual safety is maintained in spite of these differences.

As some people cope better than others with structure or lack of it, it is important that the services strike a balance between being overstructured and being unstructured. Having some structure provides a clear foundation and framework for action, but at the same time allows room to be flexible and responsive to the needs of the individual.

To be able to work within the model of care staff are required to have an openness to people using the service, many of whom are extremely vulnerable. They require support to maintain this openness and to balance it with meeting their own needs. Staff support is considered a priority at London Lighthouse, as the nature of the work can be very sad and bewildering. There is a general expectation that the support needs of each staff member and department will be addressed. The day-care staff have both individual and group support as well as professional supervision.

The day-care service staff coordinate the effective discharge of all people using the service through a joint planning meeting, including the service users, their personal carers, other service-providing departments at London Lighthouse, and external agencies if appropriate. These meetings are used to review the future need for services in order to ensure that people using them maintain an independent lifestyle and an improved quality of life.

Before agreeing a discharge date with the service user, day-care service staff confirm arrangements for other services. Follow-up visits by a key worker are organized in accordance with the discharge arrangements agreed at the planning meetings and a follow-up support group is available for people who have left the service.

QUALITY INDICATORS

Quality indicators, which measure service provision at all healing levels, are extremely important (Sumpter *et al.*, 1993). The service uses a support matrix (Norbeck, 1981) to evaluate the effectiveness of care and estimate workloads for individual workers and the whole service. The matrix measures both the intensity and duration of support required on all four levels of healing – emotional, physical, mental and spiritual.

User satisfaction is measured through a questionnaire, a consultative forum and individual reviews. Standards of care and confidentiality provided by the staff and volunteers are monitored through a combination of peer review, management supervision and staff appraisal schemes. Statistical records are maintained as part of the commitment to measuring equality of opportunity and accessibility of service provision.

A framework for measuring quality is being developed for use across the organization so that there is a more systematic approach to the setting and maintaining of standards.

There is always a need to balance the various and varied interests of all the people involved in the service, i.e. the stakeholders. The interested groups may have different value systems, therefore some consensus has to be agreed on what is meant by quality before any objectives are set. Participation is then sought from the various groups in the decisions on planning and designing services; setting standards; implementation; measuring and monitoring; analysis, review and action.

CONCLUSION

The model of care outlined above tries to explain some of the values on which the day-care service is based, with the weight of decision making being firmly with the person with HIV. The model is flexible enough to be transferable to many nursing settings. Nursing in HIV/AIDS has to adapt to change and, while doing so, be able to identify what values are important and how to maintain those values to ensure a high level of quality care.

In the current climate of change, there must be good, clear communication between all interested groups in service provision and a balance between all the various needs. Some of the issues that arise from the debates are:

- the need to protect self-referrals and self advocacy;
- the need to encourage and support people living with HIV to manage their own care packages;
- the importance of working closely with purchasers in assessing need.

The author wishes to thank all staff and service users of the Day Care Unit, London Lighthouse.

REFERENCES

Adler, M. W. (1987) Care for patients with HIV infection and AIDS. *British Medical Journal*, **295**, 27–30.

Norbeck, J. S. (1981) A model for clinical research and application. *Advances in Nursing Science*, July, 43–59.

Ryan, C. (1991) Developing a Nursing Model for Use with People with AIDS who have Neurological Involvement. Paper given at the Second European Conference for Nurses in AIDS Care, Amsterdam, 1991.

Sumpter, J., Ryan, C. and Holmes-Smith, S. (1993) HIV/AIDS: body and soul. *Nursing Times*, **89**(23), 42–5.

Families – responding to need

10

Part a: The twentieth-century family and HIV

Tony Harrison

INTRODUCTION

The family, like most conceptual entities, has never had a single, universally agreed definition. The family has evolved within and been influenced by changing structures and environments. Context, culture and challenge created a diversity of family systems, which took distinct forms in distinct geographical areas, particularly those isolated by water. National family systems evolved and acquired a heterogeneity which became established as the norm. Yet even this coalescing form continued to evolve. Wenger and Anderson (1989) chart the evolution of the family, from its agriculture-orientated large nebulous form, through the decline of the extended family in the industrial era to the modern nuclear family.

However, even this later form continues to evolve. While the stereotypical heterosexual two-parent family remains the majority, the diversity of family make-ups in terms of single parents of either gender, same-sex couples and cooperative living etc., may be seen as a challenge to this stereotype. Bor *et al.* (1993) point out that HIV may already challenge traditional definitions of the family. The stereotype of the family in the social mind always includes small children, but families remain families, albeit changing ones, regardless of the age of their children.

The popular stereotype image of the family has important implications for the provision of health care. A narrow view can lead to an initial negative response to families of differing make-ups; it can result in failure to recognize the familial needs of a client whose family differs from the norm, or in the assumption of family allegiance based on bloodline, which may not be the case from the client's point of view.

Whall (1990) gives an excellent working definition of family as: 'A self-identified group of two or more individuals whose association is characterized by special terms, who may or may not be related by bloodlines, but who function in such a way that they consider themselves to be a family'.

Families who might be defined as diverse in nature, such as gay couples, have to date borne a heavy toll within the HIV pandemic. However, the movement of the disease into the generic population is bringing the disease to the realm of the traditional family, and the work of nurses in all disciplines who have cared for these families is acknowledged in the experience of those who have received care. The incidence of HIV infection in children follows closely the incidence in women, vertical infection being the major route by which children acquire HIV, accounting for 70–80% of paediatric infection (since the treatment of blood products commenced in the UK in 1985, limiting new infections by this route in children requiring blood products) (WHO, 1991). Those children who were infected by blood products are described accurately but rather disturbingly as a 'finite group'. Given that since October 1985 blood products in the UK are both tested and heat treated, which will ensure that HIV transmission via blood products will diminish in this country, the phrase is accurate, but it is unacceptable to dismiss the substantial group of infected children in the UK with blood disorders who have received and are receiving excellent and skilled nursing intervention from the numerous haemophilia centres across the UK (Shaw, 1991). The almost familial model of such centres' care, with a resident doctor, social worker and nurse, has ensured a level of support and nursing intervention unparalleled in the infected population of children without blood disorders.

The alienation many of these families feel with regard to existing HIV-related services for those who acquired the infection by other routes has resulted in haemophilia nurses and counsellors providing total holistic support services for their own client groups throughout the UK.

Children with AIDS were first identified in Europe in 1984, although the reported numbers in the UK remain relatively small to date (delay in diagnosis associated with ignorance of HIV symptomatology in children should be taken into account). However, given recent studies of anonymous testing of neonates in the London area that show a prevalence of 1 in 500 and increasing rates of infection in women, even given that rates are consistently higher in the capital, it is fair to assume that we await a potential wave of infected and affected families over the next decade, a wave that cannot be avoided since it will consist of those already infected becoming symptomatic.

Owing to its method of transmission, HIV disease can be the sort of disease which can be shared with more than one member of the family. Multiple infection within family units brings unique problems as family members move along health continua at different times in relation to each other. This may give rise to well parents with sick children, sick parents with well children, sick parents with sick children, and so on.

The potential meeting of the family with HIV disease can occur prenatally. Today, families planning children do so with the knowledge that HIV disease exists and can be an issue for them. Similarly, the family for whom HIV is already a reality may also plan children, and require support and advice in common with all families about the risks involved. The family planning nurse/practice nurse thus becomes a vital information resource and therefore requires training for this role. In particular, Richardson (1992) highlights the needs for the reproductive rights of HIV-positive women to be protected. Nurses should therefore be educated to ensure that they provide 'full and appropriate counselling and information which respects their right to parent children' (Richardson, 1992).

The family with children and HIV disease challenges our notions of care. The unique needs of children in relation to health-care services have been the subject of several major reports (Platt, 1959; Court, 1976), the latest of which – which will hopefully prove more influential in terms of action than the two preceding it – is the Audit Commission Report (1993). These reports highlighted the needs of children for specifically trained staff, appropriate care environments and the involvement of the family in their care. Family-centred care has evolved as a basic precept of paediatric care, but this concept has remained hazy and ill defined, although some authors have recently commenced a defining process (Campbell and Summersgill, 1993); indeed, the Audit Commission revealed that this lack of definition meant that many families supposedly receiving family-centred care did not realize it.

Family-centred care seeks the involvement of the family in the care of their child in order to avoid the well-documented effects of separation/hospitalization. However, the family where the parents are ill may be incapable of such involvement, and indeed may only be able to support their child by their presence, which means that they should be in an environment where their care needs can be met at the same time as those of their child.

Such truly family-centred services are rare outside family behavioural therapy units, and yet if such care environments cannot be provided separation is inevitable, with damaging consequences. Some specialist health-care units are evolving services of a family nature, notably London Lighthouse, Mildmay Mission Hospital and The Hospital for Sick Children; the two former have child health nurses and those specializing in play on their staff in order to provide for children resident with their sick parents; Mildmay has recently completed its new unit for families and children, and The Hospital for Sick Children has for some time run a joint adult–child outpatient clinic where families can be seen together (Duggan, 1993), as have St Mary's and other London hospitals. The question must be, how can this become reality for generic non-specialist services?

This situation is pertinent not only to health but also to social services. The provision of care for children whose parents are incapacitated by ill health (in particular, HIV-related disease of the central nervous system may lead to a loss of ability to parent) has led to the development of various day-care services and the possibility of residential family services (Skinner, 1991), while others have detailed shared care arrangements (Jackson, 1992). The Department of Health has published excellent guidelines for developing services for children and families, which has now been distributed to social services departments nationally (DoH, 1992).

The family with asymptomatic disease requires support and assistance to maintain its health and to cope with the problems of living in anticipation of ill health at some indeterminate time. Positive interventions can maintain health (Lang, 1993): health visitors, with their existing links with each family in the UK, can provide this support and advice, provided they receive appropriate training about both adult and paediatric HIV disease. The creation of supportive frameworks for future use, with full consent and involvement of the family, is vital, and in particular the involvement of paediatric community nurses may be of great value; Butz *et al.* (1992) point to the value of paediatric nurse-practitioner outreach in identifying early medical problems and in providing a coordinating link between community and acute services for HIV-positive families. Many health visitors, and members of the all-too-few paediatric community nurse teams, are gaining experience and expertise in this area as well as in the area of health promotion to uninfected families.

Issues of support for both symptomatic and asymptomatic families which are holistic rather than fragmented in nature are discussed by Melvin and Sherr (1993). The vital need for support at all stages of the disease is hampered by the numbers presently involved, their geographical spread and the perceived incompatibility of families who may have received their infection by various routes. This has resulted in specialist centres providing specialist support (The Hospital for Sick Children has a nurse counsellor for HIV-positive children and their families, for example). Voluntary sector involvement (Positively Women, The Terrence Higgins Trust and Grandma's are some examples of organizations in which nurses have been moving forces) has provided excellent support services in some areas, but health-care professionals need to assess how they will provide support for increasing populations of infected families now. Models from the USA may assist in this (Crandles *et al.*, 1992). The question of voluntary sector organizations filling roles which are inadequately covered by statutory ones is one that must concern us increasingly in a health-care system exposed to market forces and their financial requirements.

The realities of the HIV pandemic highlight several distinct groupings of families with children who will require differing interventions, and it is vital that health visitors and nurses acknowledge and announce the fact that they possess many of the skills these families require in order to maintain or return them to health. The experience of the author in paediatric nurse education suggests that the mystique-laden diagnosis of HIV/AIDS in children erroneously deskills child health nurses. The perception that they do not possess the skills to provide health-care intervention for these families leads these individuals to doubt their abilities in the face of the fear of AIDS, despite the fact that they have demonstrated them frequently. The skills required to nurse the child with pneumonia remain pertinent for the HIV-positive child admitted with pneumonia: the focus of education within this field must centre on recognizing and evolving existing skills and widening knowledge bases. The response of the profession to this need for education and empowerment has been a positive one. The formation of the Paediatric AIDS Special Interest Group within the Paediatric Society of the Royal College of Nursing in early 1990, in order to group nurses who had experience of caring for children and families to share experience and support one another while being a resource for other child health nurses, was indicative of this positive approach (nursing involvement and representation within the National Forum on AIDS and Children, a body recently set up by the National Children's Bureau, continues this dissemination of nurses' experience and cross-pollinization of knowledge from other fields). If the profession's confidence to care is not realized, then other professionals will fill the gap, so denying the family faced with HIV the therapeutic intervention of nursing.

Paediatric nurse education has responded to this challenge in several centres: the Institute for Advanced Nurse Education was the first to run the ENB 934 course (Care and Management of Individuals with HIV and AIDS) focusing specifically on children's and young people's issues. Although this course is no longer available, the Charles West College of Nursing at The Hospital for Sick Children, Great Ormond Street, has recently received validation to run it and is working towards an advanced course for child health professional in HIV/AIDS in the near future. The need for such specialist courses has been represented to the ENB AIDS Education Advisory Group by the author and has been well received.

THE WELL FAMILY, AS YET UNWORRIED

HIV poses a significant threat to the health of all people, and the evolution of the pandemic has led to the societal response of scapegoating. This has led to the creation, in the public as well as the professional mind, of 'high-risk groups'. The logic of such a response, ingrained in the emotion of the masses, is inescapable. If HIV disease happens only to specific groups to which the majority do not belong, then for that majority there is little need to worry. The consequence of such a response in health education terms is obvious: those not identified as belonging to 'high-risk groups' fail to consider that they may be at risk.

The predominantly heterosexual world of the traditional twentieth-century family has so categorized itself as a low-risk group, that many health education interventions have failed to reach this target group. The Health Education Authority modified its approaches to highlight the risk for this group, but many continue in a relatively false sense of security. Media and Government pronouncements that HIV remains predominantly a problem for those in the so-called high-risk groups simply confirm this belief, which in the author's opinion may ultimately result in an increase in HIV infection for the traditional family and a reduction in commitment to health promotion approaches to this group.

The aim is not, of course, to make the family as yet unworried worry: rather, it is to highlight to all families and potential families how to maintain sexual health and avoid HIV infection. The targets for sexual health (Department of Health, 1993) put forward by the present

Government purport to advocate such health promotion: it is up to the profession to take this opportunity and make it work.

The health visitor's contact with the family places this member of the primary health-care team in an ideal position to undertake education for sexual health and HIV prevention with all families. However, the skills required for this should not be presumed to preexist: education in sexual health facilitation skills will be needed by many, although many health visitors do possess these skills and are using them to good effect.

The health visitor may also interface with the school environment for such education; however, the main thrust of education, whether direct or indirect, in terms of facilitation of sexual health education given by teachers, rests with the school nurse (Claxton, 1991). Children attending school not only comprise members of existing families but are also the embryonic members of tomorrow's families; they are therefore a primary group for HIV education in order to avoid the continuation of this pandemic.

The reality of sexual activity, HIV disease and the young requires that children have access to sexual health education which is pertinent, relevant and understandable. It is important to note that education regarding the biological aspects and pathogenesis of HIV infection is not essentially designed to bring about safer sexual behaviour.

Teachers are realistically constrained by many factors: the directives of the Government (notably Section 28 of the Local Government Act, which forbids the promotion of homosexuality as an alternative lifestyle, which has resulted in many teachers avoiding the subject altogether), their school governors and their own role. Primary health-care team members, however, are less constrained and so may be able to approach such education in conjunction with teachers in a more effective manner. Such direct educational approaches can also be augmented by nurses facilitating approaches such as cascade peer education: teaching young people to teach their own peers, whether in school or social settings. Such approaches have proved effective in the USA. Interventions by health-care workers to university and college environments through campus clinics provide similar health promotion for a population of young people who may be planning their own families. Examples of such school-based interventions, both abroad (Dibb and Warwick, 1992) and in the UK (NAT, 1991) provide templates for multidisciplinary approaches to health education which are being incorporated into their work by many school nurses.

Child health professionals encounter children and families in a range of situations: families attending child development units, families receiving nursing care in acute or outpatient units for reasons other than

HIV, all of which present opportunities for education and health enhancement. This is not to suggest that nurses providing care for the child undergoing tonsillectomy should prioritize HIV education within that setting, but rather that nurses acknowledge and be prepared for parents and children approaching them for information on either HIV or sexual health. The nurse is seen by many as a source of information on all health-care matters, and the nurse who has established a good relationship with the child and family in their care may find that parents and/or children feel empowered to discuss matters which they might find embarrassing to discuss with others. Such 'golden' opportunities should not be missed.

The individual approaches of nurses and health visitors can be very effective in empowering individuals to approach their sexual lives with confidence and safety. However, national initiatives such as Government campaigns and utilization of the media as a vehicle for information transport cannot be underestimated. Child health professionals need to ensure, through their professional bodies (Health Visitors' Association, Association of British Paediatric Nurses, Royal College of Nursing etc.), that the needs of their specific client group for health promotion are being met.

THE AFFECTED FAMILY

The growing incidence of HIV infection ensures that there are large numbers of individuals who, although not themselves infected with HIV, are affected because others they know are infected. The range of such scenarios is immense, but can be divided into secondary and primary relationships. Secondary relationships are those between individuals who are important to each other but in a less intense manner than with primary relationships; they include friends, non-immediate family members and colleagues. Primary relationships are those with parents, siblings, lovers and close friends. Both groupings may require both support and advice for themselves, and assistance in providing appropriate support for their loved one. A range of individuals may fulfil this role, but it is likely that those involved with the care of the infected individual will themselves encounter those health-care professionals involved in that person's care, thus making the nurse concerned one of the most accessible and convenient people to approach. Research into the needs of this group is currently being undertaken by Barnardo's (Orr, 1994).

The intensity and possibility of interventions for such individuals will obviously relate to the nature of the relationship between the parties concerned: those with primary relationships will need to be included in all aspects of care (subject to the patient's consent and desire), which will be detailed next; however, the needs of the affected who do not fall into this category are also of importance.

THE INFECTED FAMILY

Infected family members require primary care input from nursing professionals. Infected children receive nursing care from either specific specialist centres, such as those at The Hospital for Sick Children, London, and the City Hospital, Edinburgh, or from children's hospitals which specialize in a range of paediatric disorders, or from district general paediatric units or a combination of any of the above.

The discussion as to whether children who have HIV disease should be nursed in specialist dedicated units or within mainstream paediatric care has much in common with the similar debate in regard to adult care, and indeed interfaces with that discussion at the point at which we must consider how the principles of family-centred care can be best fulfilled when both adult and child members of a family require inpatient care (a model presently being addressed at the Mildmay Mission Hospital).

Dedicated units, such as Mildmay, may be the answer for providing joint care, as this situation is unlikely to be raised with regard to any other disease process, and certainly nursing and health visiting staff at both the specialist centres mentioned earlier have built up a vast experience of caring for such families, both in hospital and in the community, a resource which is available through the advisory capacities of both institutions and the Institute of Child Health (London) and the Paediatric AIDS Resource Centre (Edinburgh). Child health nurses should utilize such experience and willing help.

However, for the sick child with well parents (infected or not), is a specialist unit required? The author's experience of teaching paediatric nurses throughout the UK would suggest that many of them consider that the specialist care model denies both the nurse the experience of nursing children and families with HIV disease, and so the opportunity to expand skills in this area, and the child and family the integration into existing local health networks which can meet their needs without the undue disturbance associated with travel to specialist centres and with a sensitive knowledge of local amenities and environments. The answer would appear to be to offer such families a choice of care settings (particularly appreciating that those who are infected may not wish to use local services, where they could encounter friends and acquaintances who are coincidentally using other services). For this multioption model, however, several things are required:

- the establishment, already undertaken by some of the institutions mentioned above, of consultative communication with the specialist centres offering advice and support for clinical nursing management of children in local units (recommendations similar to those given by Thornes (1992));
- cross-referral arrangements (in particular with regard to intra-trust and intra-authority funding; this becomes particularly important in the reality of the loss of 'ring-fenced' AIDS monies, i.e. monies allocated specifically for HIV/AIDS care) between specialist and local centres;
- cross-referral from specialist centres to primary care teams within the families' home area (this necessitates in particular the evolution of paediatric community nurse teams as recommended by the Audit Commission (1993);
- the willingness of child health nurses to accept that HIV is a reality for their care group population, and that they have many existing skills that could be beneficially adapted to the needs of families;
- the willingness of educational establishments to provide appropriate education for such child health nurses on matters pertaining to their own field of practice (particularly as symptomatology and significance are not identical in adult and paediatric HIV disease);
- finally, a commitment to refining what Mawn et al. (1994) term an 'evolving model'.

Some child health nurses and adult nursing teams already are instituting such measures in order to provide a quality service to HIV-positive families, but this can hardly be said to be the norm or the majority. Preparatory work remains clouded by the rather short-sighted view of small identified groups of infected children clustered around specialist centres, leading to the 'not a problem here' approach to planning.

The family today is faced with the reality of a world in which HIV disease exists. The nurses who serve the needs of these families need also to face that reality for themselves as families. The process has begun, but we have far to go yet and we should start now!

REFERENCES

Audit Commission (1993) *Children First: A Study of Hospital Services*, HMSO, London.

Bor, R., Elford, J., Hart, G. and Sherr, L. (1993) The family and HIV disease. *AIDS Care*, 5(1), 3.

Butz, A., Stephenson, H., Hutton, N. *et al.* (1992) Care of HIV risk infants. Nursing outreach by PNPs. *Journal of Paediatric Health Care*, 6(3), 138–45.

Campbell, S. and Summersgill, P. (1993) Keeping it in the family. *Child Health*, **1**(1), 17–20.

Claxton, R. (1991) The school nurse's role with regard to children with HIV infection, in *Caring for Children with HIV/AIDS*, (eds R. Claxton and T. Harrison), Edward Arnold, London, pp. 119–25.

Court, S.M.D. (1976) *Fit for the Future. Report of the Committee on Child Health Services*, HMSO, London.

Crandles, S., Sussman, A., Berthaud, M. and Sunderland, A. (1992) Development of a weekly support group for caregivers of children with HIV disease. *AIDS Care*, **4**(3), 339.

Department of Health (1992) *Children and HIV. Guidelines for Local Authorities*, HMSO, London.

Department of Health (1993) *Health of the Nation Key Area Handbook: HIV and Sexual Health*, HMSO, London.

Dibb, L. and Warwick, M. (1992) Living for tomorrow. Making choices in uncertain times. HIV education in secondary schools, in *HIV/AIDS: Telling the Children*, Barnardos/Daniels Publishing, Cambridge, pp. 43–7.

Duggan, C. (1993) A family affair. Multidisciplinary care for children and families with HIV and AIDS. *Child Health*, **1**(1), 32–6.

Jackson, C. (1992) Waiting for the wave to break. *Health Visitor*, **65**(8), 262.

Lang, C. (1993) Positive steps. *Nursing Times*, **89**(11), 54.

Mawn, B., Karthas, N., Nurke, K. *et al.* (1994) Case management of the HIV positive child and family. An evolving model. *AIDS Patient Care*, **8**(2), 76–8.

Melvin, D. and Sherr, L. (1993) The child in the family. Responding to AIDS and HIV. *AIDS Care*, **5**(1), 35.

National AIDS Trust (1991) *Living for Tomorrow*, NAT, London.

Orr, N. (1994) *Research in Progress on Children and HIV in the UK*, Child AIDS No 4, National Children's Bureau, London.

Platt, H. (1959) *The Welfare of Children in Hospital*. Report of the Platt Committee. HMSO, London.

Richardson, D. (1992) Women, AIDS and reproduction. *Health Visitor*, **65**(5), 159–62.

Shaw, A. (1991) Nursing care of children with haemophilia and HIV infection, in *Caring for Children with HIV and AIDS*, (eds R. Claxton and T. Harrison), Edward Arnold, London, pp. 60–8.

Skinner, K. (1991) Social care for families affected by HIV infection, in *Caring for Children with HIV and AIDS*, (eds R. Claxton and T. Harrison), Edward Arnold, London, pp. 129–30.

Thornes, R. (1993) *Bridging the Gap*, Action for Sick Children, London.

UK Declaration Group (1990) *The UK Declaration of the Rights of People with HIV and AIDS*, London.

Wenger, A.F. and Anderson, J.J. (1989) The developing family, in *Family Centred Nursing Care of Children*, (eds Foster, Hunsberger and Anderson), W.B. Saunders, Philadelphia, pp. 49–91.

Whall, A. (1990) The family as the unit of care in nursing, in *Concepts Fundamental to Nursing*, (eds R. Ismeurt, E. Arnold and V. Carson), Stringhouses, Pennsylvania, pp. 52–7.

WHO/EC Collaborating Centre on AIDS (1991) AIDS *Surveillance in Europe. WHO Paris Quarterly Report. No 30*, p. 29.

Part b: Family care – the Mildmay Mission Hospital

Mavis Hibbard

'We are committed to holistic care and believe each person is unique in that they are spiritual, physical and psychological beings'.

INTRODUCTION

Since 1988, Mildmay Mission Hospital has been providing holistic palliative care for people infected/affected by HIV/AIDS. Initially all our patients were men, but by 1991 statistics showed that we were admitting increasing numbers of women, all of childbearing age and many already with children (Table 10.1).

Table 10.1 Mildmay Mission Hospital – female admissions (Patient Administration Statistics Mildmay Mission Hospital, 1993)

Year	Referral	Admissions
February 1988 – September 1990 (2.5 years)	9	6
October 1990 – March 1991 (6 months)	28	22
April 1991 – March 1992 (12 months)	35	28
April 1992 – December 1992	39	32

(Patient administration statistics Mildmay Mission Hospital, 1993)

The Mildmay statistics were concurrent with the Communicable Disease Report (CDR) figures. Anonymous testing in antenatal clinics during 1990–92 showed that all such clinics in London had HIV-positive women attending and that, in nearby Newham, 1–200 women attending were HIV positive. We began to receive requests to admit children with their mothers, as often they had been separated for several weeks due to either the mother or the child or both being hospitalized in an acute centre. We assisted where we could but, with an adult unit, skill mix and existing staffing levels, it soon became clear that this was not the way forward.

The Chief Executive and Directors of Mildmay studied the available statistics and projected trends, and had discussions with service users, professional and voluntary agencies and the Department of Health. In 1992 the vision was born. An appeal was launched for funds to build a family unit, which would enable families to stay together while one or more members received palliative care. The Family Care Centre opened in September 1993 – the start of a learning process.

OVERVIEW OF THE UNIT

The centre provides care on two floors with six separate rooms on each, containing all the necessary ancillary features; the ground floor is given over to a well-equipped day nursery, additional relatives/close friends accommodation and a bereavement suite.

Care is given by an interdisciplinary team comprising doctors, nurses, counsellors and social care workers, dietitians, occupational therapists, physiotherapists, community liaison nurses, nursery nurses and chaplains.

CLIENT GROUP

The largest proportion of our families come from sub-Saharan Africa and will often be far away from their extended families. They may be refugees or asylum seekers. The remainder of our families are those who have contracted the disease through substance abuse, and two Caucasian women who were infected through heterosexual sex. The majority of parents are either single or separated from their spouses; their average age is 30.4 years and the greater number of patients are women.

Families choose to use the service in different ways. Most elect to have their partner and children resident in the same room; others will elect for a partner and children to stay in the relatives' suite, while some mothers who are tired and ill and in need of a complete rest will decide that the child should stay with carers and visit daily.

One family, where both parents and one child have symptomatic disease and where the marriage is under great strain, chooses to come for respite care separately: the child resides with whoever is the patient at any given time. They feel they both get increased respite this way.

Families who use our service are often living in fear, isolation and bewilderment: when one or more members of a family have AIDS, the whole family will be affected by the major change this implies. Care for these families cannot be a symmetric package but must be flexible in order to meet their needs.

Admission to the Family Care Centre is via a referral to the community liaison nurses; referrals may be made by GPs, acute hospitals, social workers, voluntary agencies, patients or relatives. All referrals must be accompanied by an up-to-date medical statement and all patients undergo preadmission assessment by a community liaison nurse.

Mildmay is committed to patient-directed care administered by an interdisciplinary team; each discipline carries out its own patient assessment in accordance with the patient's own prioritized needs. The type of care is categorized as follows:

- respite – admission from the community;
- convalescence/rehabilitation – admission from acute hospital;
- terminal;
- long-term – more than 3 months – until death.

For an interdisciplinary team to operate successfully, the following must be attained: each individual must have a clear understanding of his or her role and boundaries; all team members must understand the roles of other disciplines and possess excellent communication skills, both verbal and written. The Family Care Centre interdisciplinary team meets three mornings a week in order to discuss and plan the care of patients; by the fourth day of admission assessments will have been made and a care plan instituted. On the seventh day a key worker is appointed who is responsible for discharge planning and liaison with community agencies. Nurses have an important role within the team as the only 24-hour caregivers who are involved with all patients, albeit to a varying degree.

PHILOSOPHY OF NURSING CARE

We are committed to holistic care and believe each person is unique as a spiritual, physical and psychological being. We believe that:

1. Each person, their carer, partner and family, has the right to be cared for equally, regardless of race, religion, lifestyle, age, sexual or political orientation. All visitors (including telephone callers) will be treated hospitably, greeted with respect, care and a friendly manner.
2. The individual living with HIV/AIDS has the right to skilled nursing care which, in the promotion of health and recovery, will help him or her to be as independent as possible, maintain his/her dignity, foster a sense of identity and assist in achieving a peaceful and pain free death.
3. Patients have the right to know how and why they are being treated and what alternatives are available. Enough information should be given so that they can make an informed decision.
4. Patients and those nominated by them, whether family, friends or partners, should be encouraged to participate in contributing towards their care.
5. Each person has access to the skill and knowledge of the multidisciplinary team, whose involvement, coordinated by both the patient and the nursing staff, determines the best outcome for the patient.
6. Mildmay aims to maintain a positive environment. Individuals with HIV/AIDS will be nursed with full respect for their individuality.
7. Spiritual support is available for patients, carers, partners and family as they search for meaning and purpose in life, suffering and loss.
8. Health education should be an integral part of the care of patients, thereby enhancing their quality of life.
9. Research, the setting, monitoring and evaluation of standards of care is an important basis for improvement of the quality of nursing practice.
10. As professionally qualified practitioners, nurses are accountable for their actions and must abide by the UKCC Code of Conduct.

MODEL OF NURSING CARE

The nurses are divided into two teams per floor, each team being responsible for three patients and their families. This will involve caring for many affected individuals. The model of nursing care for adults is flexible, as the content, interaction and needs of families may differ greatly. It is underpinned by Roper's 'Activities of daily living' (Roper, Logan and Tierney, 1990) and influenced by Orem, given that the accent at Mildmay is on self-directed care. At present we are formulating a model of care for children which is based on Casey and Mobb (1988). The 'named nurse' system is in operation in the Family Care Centre.

NURSING SKILL MIX

The factors affecting the choice of skill mix are:

- AIDS is a multisystem disease.
- The Family Care Centre cares for adults and children.
- Families using the service are multicultural.

Given the above, the skill mix needs to be diverse and must include RGNs, RMNs and RSCNs. It is advisable to appoint nurses with a knowledge of HIV/AIDS and nurses from multicultural backgrounds.

Nurses need to be flexible, as caring for families may include giving a complex regimen of intravenous drugs, reading a story to an active 3-year-old or sitting with a patient suffering from dementia.

The inclusion of RSCNs in the skill mix is essential (Audit Commission,) but these nurses must also possess general adult nursing skills. Health-care assistants are included in our skill mix but numbers are minimal.

FAMILY ISSUES

Socioeconomic factors play an essential role here: for example, adequate housing is very often a significant unmet need for refugees and asylum seekers. As with financial issues, such people lack knowledge of the UK welfare and statutory benefits system and may be hampered by their inability to communicate well in English. They also fear that knowledge of their HIV status may hinder applications for refugee status (Hamujuni, 1993). Housing, too, is often inappropriate for people suffering from chronic fatigue, weakness and mobility dysfunction.

Stigma surrounding the disease leads to fear of others knowing that they are living with AIDS which in turn leads to social isolation, fear of reprisals, and alienation by family, neighbours and statutory bodies. Some of our patients have been spat on, had graffiti sprawled over their homes, had water poured over them and been forced to move. One delightful young mother recently told the author how safe and relaxed she had felt during her stay in the centre – only her partner and professional workers knew of her and her daughter's HIV status.

Frequent hospitalization for parents and/or children gives rise to long separations and also to periods of alternative care for a child, either with a member of the extended family or with a local authority foster parent. When parents with AIDS are left to care for their children without help, extreme tiredness and weakness affects their ability to cope. Many of our families are single parents and face isolation, lack of family support and help in caring for children; for several of our mothers, their HIV status has been the cause of matrimonial breakdown.

Issues surrounding diagnosis are the cause of intense concern for families:

> Should I tell my child my diagnosis?
> Should I tell my child I am going to die?
> Should I tell my child his/her diagnosis?
> Should I tell my child he/she is going to die?
> Who will care for my child when I die?
> Who should I tell?

The issues around disclosure and child care are the most difficult and distressing for parents. Lack of extended family in this country and shortage of foster parents only increases this distress.

NURSING ISSUES

The Family Care Centre operates a model of patient-directed care in which patients are given sufficient information to make informed choices. This raises many issues for nurses:

- patients' ability to make informed decisions through clinical mental illness (multicausal) and temporary affective disorders;
- nurses' own agenda regarding life and death;
- duty of care/responsibility;
- accountability;
- pressure from family and friends.

HIV/AIDS has raised many questions for palliative care services. The ever-increasing treatments now available and the long prognosis for life have resulted in a merging of acute and palliative philosophies. A large amount of care given by palliative care services is by definition acute/curative, although this does not affect the virus itself. Where children with the disease are concerned, extra emotional pressure is brought to bear by families unwilling to let go and health-care workers reluctant to stop the fight when options, however futile, are still available.

Caring for children, well or sick, whose parents have a life-threatening disease raises more complex issues for nurses:

- Different cultures have different ideas on child care, discipline, hygiene, health and safety, play, love and affection.
- Cognitive impairment in parents may affect their decisions and abilities.

- Behavioural problems in parents – e.g. drug abuse, personality disorders, violence/aggression – will produce a desire on the part of the professional to protect the child.
- Cultural hierarchy may mean different instructions and arguments over a child's treatment – grandparents may well be dominant.
- Parents' refusal to trust or be guided by medical information and/or advice may put the child at risk of illness/infection.
- Cultural and spiritual beliefs may affect parental decisions about medical intervention and child care which opposes western beliefs.
- Child protection issues – is a child at risk when parents are using drugs while showering their child with love and affection? These parents are going to die soon.
- Adoption and fostering issues – these decisions are often left until the parent is very ill, and they can cause immense distress to all involved.

The cultural differences of African families mean that nurses have to take into account a number of factors when caring for them:

- Decision making – although the mother will be the main carer, the father has a large input into decisions concerning children.
- The shame of HIV infection is possibly greater for African families, hence confidentiality is paramount.
- The idea of palliative care may be unknown.
- Self-directed care may prove difficult for patients who would prefer professionals to make decisions, particularly around the question of when to cease active treatment.

HOW NURSES HAVE RISEN TO THE CHALLENGE

Nurses have learned to meet the challenge by treating each patient as an individual who has diverse social, medical and psychological needs, all of which deserve equal consideration and attention. Nurses have shown they are able to adapt their skills to meet the new demands made on their profession. Nurses from other ethnic groups have moved more slowly into the field of HIV/AIDS.

THE NURSERY

In March 1993, a day nursery facility was opened at Mildmay in response to parental need for respite from their children. The nursery is staffed by qualified nursery nurses. Transport is provided for children resident in three local boroughs. For other children living outside the area, three local authorities provide transport and the remainder are brought by their parents. In September 1993 the nursery became an integral part of the Family Care Centre.

The staff operate a shift system and are available to assist parents in caring for children from 8 a.m. to 8 p.m. The team works closely with the family/foster carers, the interdisciplinary team, community social workers and health visitors and members of the acute hospital teams.

The split between HIV-positive and HIV-negative children is approximately 50:50, with three of the children attending currently being symptomatic. All children attending are affected by HIV/AIDS and all are or will be bereaved of one or both parents. The nursery nurses need to be aware of sudden changes in a child's physical condition, and one of our doctors has specific responsibility for the nursery.

Behavioural problems in children whose parents have frequent hospitalizations and who themselves have frequent foster care are particularly challenging for the staff.

WHAT WE HAVE LEARNT

Although we consulted numerous professionals and voluntary workers before the centre opened, the first year has been a learning situation. For the most part, this has centred around aspects of sub-Saharan African culture, including:

- the importance of family hierarchy;
- the need to express grief freely and on their own;
- the needs of African men to communicate with male staff;
- the difficulties which African women, whose lives have been 'directed', may experience when they have the opportunity to make choices;
- the dietary needs and the emphasis placed on good nutrition throughout their illness.

Understanding the interaction within a family is vital for the provision of effective services: major changes for one member will affect the whole family unit (Melvin and Sherr, 1993). When admitting children (well or sick) with parents, it is essential to obtain a social work report prior to admission, in order to understand what are invariably complex social issues and to provide continuity of care. There is a need to know who is going to care for the child in an emergency, e.g. the transfer of a parent to an acute centre, or indeed the death of a parent.

If they are to benefit from their stay, parents must continue to assume responsibility for their 'well' children. However, the children need to be cared for by staff as much as possible, and in this respect nursery nurses have a vital role to play.

THE FUTURE

The Family Care Centre's unique model of care will continue to meet the challenge of increasing numbers of families infected/affected by HIV/AIDS. Services for families are still in their infancy, with many initiatives still in the planning stage. As community services emerge, Mildmay will continue to work alongside them, thus enabling families to continue living at home for as long as possible. The specialist expertise based in one centre, available to all families affected by AIDS, aims to enhance community care.

REFERENCES

Audit Commission (1993) *Children First: A Study of Hospital Services*. HMSO.

Casey, A. and Mobb, S. (1988) Partnership in practice: nurses and parents form a primary nursing team. *Nursing Times*, **84**(44), 67–8.

Hamujuni, B. (1993) Additional issues for refugee families – placement needs of children affected by HIV. Seminar 14–15 January 1993.

Melvin, D. and Sherr, L. (1993) The child in the family – responding to AIDS and HIV. *AIDS Care*, **5**(1), 35–42.

Roper, N., Logan, W.W. and Tierney, A.T. (1990) *The Elements of Nursing: A Model for Nursing Based on a Model of Living*, 2nd edn. Churchill Livingstone, Edinburgh.

FURTHER READING

Rutter, M. (1981a) *Maternal Deprivation Reassessed*, Penguin, Harmondsworth.

Rutter, M. (1981b) *Helping Troubled Children*, Penguin, Harmondsworth.

Sherr, L. (1991) *HIV and AIDS in Mothers and Babies*, Blackwell Scientific, Oxford.

PART THREE
Future Challenges: Expanding the Horizons

INTRODUCTION

There is no doubt that, as Dr Jonathan Mann claimed at the Tenth International Conference on AIDS in Yokohama, Japan, in August 1994, we live in an exciting and unsettling period of history in relation to the AIDS pandemic. Those who have been involved in this work for some time are now shocked when they encounter prejudice and intolerance, and stunned when they come across nurses and other health-care staff who, despite the best efforts of educationalists, remain ignorant and ill informed. However, attitudes are difficult to change, particularly towards those marginalized by society. In particular there remains much work to do with those people who fall outside even the parameters of 'a normal HIV/AIDS patient', that is, those who are not the stereotypical middle-class gay man with a good education, a job and lots of loving support. This is an image used effectively by the media and the Hollywood entertainment machine, but one which fails to describe the reality.

Even in the western world – and this is increasingly the case – millions of people lack access to appropriate health care. There is no doubt that influences of gender, low social class, unemployment, poverty, drug misuse and mental ill health not only increase vulnerability to HIV infection but also determine access to and use of health-care services.

This final section contains chapters which examine in some detail these issues of access and equity in health care, specific issues which affect the behaviour and care of drug users, and the challenge of caring for those people with HIV who manifest neurological and mental health problems. All these issues are enormous challenges for nursing staff in the future, and the manner in which the profession manages to deal with these groups, who are even further marginalized by issues other than their HIV status, will provide important lessons for nursing across the board.

Obviously it is not within the scope of a volume such as this to deal with all the global challenges posed by HIV and AIDS, and this point is made in the concluding chapter, which sets the discussion in the context of the future. It is important for all nurses to realize that traditional approaches to public health, disease prevention and the provision of care have all been changed beyond recognition by HIV and AIDS, and that many aspects of nursing will never be the same again. This is vividly demonstrated by the innovative responses used in contacting the 'hard to reach', and in making the necessary changes to services to ensure that they are 'user friendly' and not run solely for the benefit of professionals and a few 'chosen' clients. Challenges are met and innovations described in relation to providing the service which makes the most sense in terms of prevention, and in assisting the client struggling to arrive at positive life choices. Often, in spearheading these changes, nurses have had to challenge 'dogmatic' philosophical stances of agencies and organizations. This process is still vital, perhaps even more so as HIV and AIDs becomes an issue which must be embraced by the mainstream health-care service.

Reducing inequality of access and care provision for people affected by HIV/AIDS

Steve Cranfield

'The epidemiological paradox is that HIV/AIDS may become less of an issue but also more of a problem' (Bennett and Ferlie, 1994).

BRINGING HIV IN FROM THE MARGINS: CHANGING PATTERNS OF RESPONSE

In 1991 the UKCC set out a series of principles designed to underpin the aim of meeting the health-care needs of all individuals, groups and communities (UKCC, 1991). The fourth of these principles is 'the reduction in inequality of access and/or care provision'. This laudable principle has faced, and continues to face, a number of specific challenges in the context of HIV/AIDS, and this chapter sets out to explore some of the main implications of these for nurses.

Current inequalities of access are due to two main factors: the unequal distribution of HIV infection in society, and negative attitudes to those infected and insufficient awareness of their needs. Both of these can impede uptake of services or thwart initiatives designed to increase uptake. Statistics on the prevalence of HIV infection and AIDS continue to indicate the unequal distribution of cases among the population, in both demographic and geographical terms (PHLS, 1993). The current prevalence of HIV in England is focal, that is, it is not evenly distributed: there are significant variations around the country. The Thames Health Regions continue to report the majority of positive HIV tests and AIDS cases, although this may in part reflect the fact that people with HIV are rently seeking services based within these areas. Although in some reas, such as Scotland, the main source of HIV infection has been through injecting drug use, in general the first wave of infection in Britain, as in the United States, has occurred in gay and bisexual men. One consequence of this pattern of prevalence is that access to specialist diagnostic, treatment and support facilities is markedly better in some parts of the country than in others.

Varying attitudes and levels of medical and nursing expertise in dealing with HIV also mean that many people with the virus have 'voted with their feet' and moved to areas where they can be assured of respectful, prompt and reliable diagnosis and treatment. There can be little doubt that in many cases this has proved lifesaving (Kirk, 1992). However, this uneven and unequal distribution of resources and expertise has led some to want to change the situation, to ensure that the principle of equality of access set out by the UKCC becomes a reality for all in their own communities.

Access to health care is also a political and social issue. The French social scientist Michaël Pollak (1992) has argued that the rapid diffusion of HIV among marginalized groups in society – gay and bisexual men, and injecting drug users – has created problems for public policy on HIV prevention and access to service provision. At the beginning of the epidemic many governments and professional groupings played an inactive 'wait-and-see' role. In the absence of public action, there was an unprecedented mobilization against AIDS on the part of grassroots community and self-help groups and networks. The demand, in developed western countries at least, for increased access to information, treatment and social support has been largely consumer led and concentrated in major urban areas, where the incidence of infection has been highest. This has resulted in the creation of a range of specialist statutory services, staffed by dedicated teams of professionals who have developed considerable expertise. The 1980s saw a lively debate about 'specialist' versus 'generic': some argued against what they saw as the 'ghettoization' of HIV, while others pointed to the fact that, in addition to the demographic inequalities outlined above, many of those affected by HIV suffer from existing prejudice and discrimination, are not well served by the medical establishment and are hence more likely to face inequalities of access on a number of fronts. The argument for specialist centres was compelling.

In the mid-1990s we appear to have entered a new phase of the epidemic and the public response to this (Bennett and Ferlie, 1994). Professional awareness and mobilization have increased dramatically and a steadily growing number of non HIV-specialist nurses have had experience of caring for people with HIV. Early projections of the scale of the epidemic in the UK have been revised (PHLS, 1993), and while these projections are still subject to several major uncertainties, they are now considerably reduced. As a result HIV is no longer being perceived as a new or unfamiliar disease. The move is to mainstream HIV services and bring them in from the margins, thereby removing their special status. They are thus increasingly having to compete with other items on the health-care, social and economic agenda. The implications of this process for reducing inequalities of access to care have yet to be determined.

In the changing political and economic climate, reducing inequalities of access prompts a number of important professional, ethical and economic questions. Given the costs of HIV treatment alone, is equal access for all at all stages of HIV infection a realistic option (assuming, of course, that everyone is aware of his or her own antibody status)? Much as practitioners may cherish the primacy of the notion of responding to need, who decides which needs are legitimate? Is it inevitable that hard-nosed economic decisions will need to be taken about who gets which kind of treatment and at what stage? And how do we tackle negative attitudes to people with HIV among health-care colleagues (which may include complaints of favouritism, patient-coddling and special treatment) that still impede access to and uptake of heath care, especially among marginalized groups?

Nurses have a pivotal role to play in influencing the development of the debate about access in the context of HIV/AIDS. This chapter looks at access to statutory health-care provision for HIV, and explores some of the emerging issues brought about by specific developments in diagnosis and treatment; it then identifies the implications for nurses and suggests strategies for reducing inequalities of access in the increasingly entrepreneurial environment in which health care is allocated and delivered.

NURSES AND ACCESSIBILITY

Probably few would take issue with the argument that nurses, by the very nature of their role, are more accessible to patients and clients, and perhaps more trusted by them, than other health-care professionals. Sadly, however, examples of prejudice and discrimination against people affected by HIV are not hard to come by in the nursing literature (Irwin, 1992; Rose and Platzer, 1993) or in personal accounts of care written by people with HIV themselves (Madeley, 1987):

'I was awoken by the sound of rustling plastic and opened my eyes to be confronted by a nurse in boots, plastic apron, hat and rubber gloves. I wanted to die there and then. When she returned 20 minutes later I asked why she was dressed in this weird outfit and was told she had the right to protect herself. I replied that I also had a choice and I chose not to be cared for by an ill-informed and insensitive nurse.'

Examples like the above should not, however, obscure the fact that individual nurses and nursing organizations were among the first to begin to listen to people with AIDS and to respond to grassroots pressures for improved access to prevention and treatment. The development of many innovative HIV-specific services was one of the nursing success stories of the 1980s. This has been especially the case in such key areas as community and peer education, low threshold services and outreach. Nurses continue to play an important role in helping to develop and sustain new models of health promotion and HIV prevention, particularly those targeted at groups of people frequently seen as hard to reach: injecting drug users; young people; people of minority ethnic groups; women and men working in the sex industry; travellers; and homeless people. Examples of nursing-led initiatives can be found in site-based and peripatetic health-care teams in both urban and rural areas (Datt and Feinmann, 1990; McGuiness and Knight, 1991), outreach work with the young, the homeless and women prostitutes (Thomson, 1991) and in easy-access centres for drug users coming into contact with the criminal justice system (Coleman *et al.*, 1989). These continue to open up unique opportunities for health education and treatment.

Often improved accessibility is achieved not by increased resources or innovation in services but by changes in organization and administration. Nurses, because of their relative closeness to the client, are often uniquely placed to spot ways in which the system can be made more accessible, efficient, or work more beneficially for the client. Take the fairly common problem of multiple outpatient appointments, for example. People with HIV frequently have several time-consuming appointments in a variety of departments, sometimes on different sites. The time, forbearance and personal organization this requires may be off-putting to many, especially those with child-care or work commitments or a less than totally organized lifestyle. Attacking the problem of non-attendance and dropout rates is vital to keep people in touch with helping services, to help support behaviour change and provide medical follow-up (Strang, 1990). As a result, many outpatient and genitourinary medicine (GUM) clinics and drug services have adopted a more 'user friendly' approach. Access, uptake and patient retention have been improved by such strategies as combining HIV medical and drug treatment appointments (Brettle *et al..*, 1992), integrating HIV paediatric and adult outpatient services (Hutchinson and Kurth, 1991; Mok, 1991), or by incorporating aspects of 'customer care' to make services more responsive and attractive.

An area where nursing strategies have excelled to date is low threshold services. These aim to attract people to seek help by minimizing obstacles to treatment (such as rules for compliance); most have an open-door policy. One of the most successful examples of this approach has been the establishment of needle exchange programmes (Stimson *et al.*, 1988), in which nurses, not unsurprisingly, usually make up the majority of staff (Lart and Stimson, 1990). The majority of these services are perceived as user friendly and have succeeded in attracting injectors not in contact with other helping agencies, and many provide a wide range of health and support services in addition to clean injecting equipment and risk-reduction advice. Significantly, those pilot exchanges which were perceived as inaccessible by clients (owing to reduced opening times, or being located in remote districts) quickly closed. For many drug users the exchange proves to be a conduit into GUM, contraceptive and antenatal services, general medical care and HIV follow-up: services that can all too easily prove inaccessible to clients because of their drug-using lifestyle (Carvell and Hart, 1990).

Low threshold services with an HIV/AIDS component are not limited to those aimed at drug users. Others target women, homeless people, those with alcohol use problems and the mentally ill. Acknowledging the value of such services, the government's White Paper *Health of the Nation* (Department of Health, 1992a) has suggested that they be extended to young people seeking contraceptive help and advice. The accompanying key area handbook also recommends setting up 'drop-in' clinics with a no-appointment system at health centres and GP practices (Department of Health, 1993).

HIV ANTIBODY TESTING

Since 1985 the HIV antibody test has been made publicly available on a voluntary basis, to encourage people to come forward for testing if they think they have been at risk of infection and to receive counselling, support and medical aftercare. Testing is a cornerstone of Government HIV prevention policies, although calls for compulsory testing have so far been resisted, whether in relation to 'high-risk' groups such as gay men, injecting drug users, prostitutes and prisoners, or to the general population.

In the UK, the majority of HIV antibody testing is carried out through GUM clinics. Anecdotal evidence suggests that some people, including women, members of minority ethnic groups and younger gay men, may be reluctant to attend these settings and do not wish to discuss their anxieties with, or request a test from, their family doctor. Many people would prefer to attend a clinic separate from other services. In 1992, the UK Government issued guidance on establishing additional sites for HIV antibody testing (Department of Health, 1992b). A proposed aim is to enable earlier diagnosis of HIV infection and improve access to medical care and follow-up. However, the benefits of early diagnosis for individual health have been called into question following research findings into early intervention treatments (see below).

In many countries innovative programmes have been set up to make voluntary antibody testing more accessible in a variety of different settings, e.g. needle exchanges, antenatal clinics, peripatetic health-care teams, prisons, bath houses and saunas. But nearly all of these programmes to date have been targeted at perceived high-risk groups: gay and bisexual men, pregnant women, injecting drug users, prisoners, and women and men working in the sex industry. It remains to be seen whether alternative testing sites will reach those who consider they might have been infected but who are put off by current services, as opposed to the 'worried well', for want of a better term. It does not necessarily follow that increased *availability* of the test will result in improved *accessibility* to those most at risk. There may be lessons to be drawn here from the limited success of similar initiatives in the United States during the 1980s:

> '...the use of the traditional STD [sexually transmitted disease] clinic as a model for the new test sites, coupled with financial stringency on the basis of government cost–benefit analysis, severely curtailed the counselling activities of the alternative testing sites....[An increase in] demands for testing legitimized testing over counselling, education or community awareness – though all of these had been proven to influence the meaning and consequences of test taking' (Patton, 1990).

In 1991 preliminary results of the Department of Health's anonymized serosurveys indicated that 1 in 500 pregnant women attending certain antenatal clinics in London were HIV antibody-positive, with a prevalence of between 1 in 200 and 1 in 1000 in those London districts participating in the study (Department of Health, 1992a). In 1992 the Department issued guidelines for offering voluntary named HIV antibody testing to women receiving antenatal care, with the aim of making the test and appropriate counselling more available to pregnant women, especially in areas of known higher incidence of HIV infection (Department of Health, 1992c).

Current guidelines stress the need to build in safeguards to ensure the confidential and voluntary nature of the test. Certain concerns inevitably arise, however. The guidelines state that 'the test must only be performed with the woman's explicit consent obtained after appropriate pretest discussion in private'. But how are such prerequisites as privacy, confidentiality and explicit consent to be met in the case of, say, an anxious teenage woman attending a busy clinic for her first appointment, accompanied by her mother or partner, neither of whom knows about her previous risk behaviour? How much time do midwives and obstetricians have to provide adequate information, risk-reduction advice and counselling? Some antenatal clinics have attempted to solve these problems by sending the prospective mother information about HIV and the test in advance, but it has yet to be established how helpful or effective this is, either as a health education tool or as a means of preparing women for counselling about the test.

CONTINUING CARE FOR PEOPLE WITH HIV OR AIDS

A wide range of potential services should be accessible to people with HIV and AIDS if they are to function in their own communities. These include:

- hospital-based and community nursing;
- various home therapies (intravenous, nutritional and physical);
- advice and assistance on finance and legal needs;
- dental care;
- drug dependency treatment;
- individual, group and family counselling;
- housing;
- day care and volunteer support for help with the activities of daily living, such as cooking, shopping and cleaning;
- transport;
- help with claiming benefits for which they may be eligible.

The list goes on. Clearly, the resource implications are enormous. Recent and future developments in medical diagnosis and treatment are likely to have a profound impact on pressures for access to these resources and forms of support.

DEVELOPMENTS IN DIAGNOSIS

A number of tests are available, or being developed, which indicate the state and functioning of the immune system in people with HIV infection (Masur, 1990; Bowman, 1991). Some of these laboratory tests may have a predictive value, that is, they may indicate susceptibility to disease progression in advance of the appearance of physical signs and symptoms. Tests are either HIV-specific (e.g. p24 antigen and antibody) or non HIV-specific (e.g. CD4 count, β_2 microglobulin and cytomegalovirus antibody). Although none of these tests in isolation gives a total picture of immune functioning, taken together they can provide important information and may play a significant part in the clinical management of HIV infection as a chronic illness. However, acceptance of the validity and usefulness of these tests is far from universal. Some are still in the experimental stage and many physicians are sceptical of their validity and reliability, and of the cost of using them (Project Inform, 1991). For the time being, access to many tests with predictive values is likely to be restricted to people attending specialist HIV treatment centres and those taking part in clinical trials.

How routine will these tests become? Offering them on a regular basis is costly and may provide conflicting or limited information about the course of individual infection; they may create more or less uncertainty. Clinicians may speculate on how beneficial or cost-effective this is for people with HIV who are currently well. On the other hand, in the absence of such tests it is hard to see how preventive treatments are to be effectively targeted at those most at risk of developing symptomatic infection (which may be more cost-effective in the long run, as well as beneficial for the individual). It has been argued that informing people of their results requires specialist counselling (in addition, that is, to pre- and post-test counselling) to help them understand the meaning of the results and to deal with the many anxieties and concerns this can raise (Miller *et al.* 1991). This clearly has additional resource implications which may further limit the availability and accessibility of such tests, or the confidence of staff in using them.

EARLY INTERVENTION AND CLINICAL TRIALS

Early intervention is a term used to refer to therapies against HIV for people with asymptomatic infection. These therapies may prevent some diseases and delay the onset of others. Any early intervention fits into one of three possible approaches: antivirals, e.g. zidovudine (AZT); immune stimulants, e.g. postexposure vaccine and α-interferon; and opportunistic infection prevention, e.g. the prophylactic use of pentamidine and co-trimoxazole (Septrin). As with laboratory tests with predictive values, some of the more recent treatments are at the experimental stage and likely to be restricted to those attending specialist HIV treatment centres or enrolled in clinical trials. The question as to whether people have the 'right' of access to experimental treatments is a controversial one, raising many profound ethical, professional, legal and economic dilemmas.

It has been argued that early intervention will come to be the mainstay of HIV treatment (Francis *et al.*, 1991). However, caution continues to be urged: some treatments may have limited or no use and may lead to viral resistance. The findings of the large-scale multicentre Concorde-1 trial have called into doubt the value of AZT in preventing disease progression in people with asymptomatic infection (Concorde Coordinating Committee, 1994). Even among people aware of their positive status, knowledge of the possible benefits of early intervention is not widespread. In San Francisco, for example, where there is already a high level of community awareness about AIDS, one study found that a substantial proportion of people with HIV seek help only late in their disease progression, do not know their CD4 count and have only limited access to health care (Katz *et al.*, 1991). Despite the high profile of HIV in contemporary life, there is clearly much to be done in promoting increased uptake of vital diagnostic measures and available treatments.

It is perhaps not surprising that many groups are consistently underrepresented in early intervention treatment trials, including women, ethnic minorities, injecting drug users, people with mental illness, those in prison and people who are homeless or unemployed: all groups, in fact, which are traditionally underserved in terms of health care (Besch *et al.*, 1991). These groups tend to present for treatment later in the disease progression (Mays and Cochran, 1991; Schoenbaum and Webber, 1991) and have higher dropout rates (Arici *et al.*, 1991).

Special considerations may apply to some children with HIV. In the United States there have been difficulties in establishing the rights of children with HIV in foster care to be allowed access to clinical trials because of concerns for their rights and safety. Some clinicians have argued that the inclusion of any children in treatment protocols represents 'an intrusion into a group of vulnerable subjects' (Quaggin, 1987). There have also been legal complications over giving and obtaining consent by proxy (Martin and Sacks, 1990). In the UK guidance on children and HIV issued by the Department of Health (1992d) to local authorities does not yet offer specific advice on consent to treatment among children in care, and this remains a complex area.

CHANGING DEFINITIONS OF AIDS

One of the most interesting factors affecting access to care and treatment is the changing medical definition of AIDS itself. The most widely used current definition of HIV infection and AIDS is that used by the Public

Health Centers for Disease Control (CDC) in Atlanta, Georgia, USA. This definition has undergone a number of changes. Currently AIDS is diagnosed by the presence of certain defined indicator diseases, such as toxoplasmosis, *Pneumocystis carinii* pneumonia and candidiasis (CDC, 1987). Eligibility for anti-HIV treatments and access to welfare benefits and other forms of social support require, in most instances, a specific HIV-related diagnosis. Access to treatment and care, therefore, largely depends on the knowledge and diagnostic capabilities of individual physicians. Where HIV-related expertise is lacking, as in many prisons or areas of known low incidence of infection, people with symptomatic HIV infection may go undiagnosed and untreated.

The CDC definition has been criticized as failing to take into account differences in the presentation of HIV infection, especially among women and members of ethnic minorities (Patton, 1990). This led to calls for an extension of the case definition to include the level of CD4 counts and such conditions as pulmonary tuberculosis, recurrent pneumonia and invasive cervical cancer. Such changes have been incorporated in the revised US case definition after protracted public debate (CDC, 1992). The most recent (1993) European AIDS surveillance Case Definition includes the three new indicator diseases mentioned above but not levels of CD4 cell count (WHO/EC, 1993).

Many have welcomed the potential widening of the health-care 'net'. Redefining AIDS may result in increasing the availability of vital care and support services to a greater number of people in need. But it could also be argued that this is essentially a displacement activity: how we define and refine our definitions of the syndrome may be important, but what really needs to change is a health-care system which reflects and possibly perpetuates social inequalities. More to the point, no publicly funded health-care and welfare system is at present likely to be able to meet the needs of ever-increasing numbers of people requesting additional benefits and costly forms of treatment and social support. To avoid being overwhelmed, any system will simply raise the threshold of access by changing its eligibility criteria. Redefining AIDS may not provide a long-term solution to demands for equality of access since it may result in further and more elaborate restrictions on access to treatment.

REDUCING INEQUALITIES OF ACCESS: NURSING DILEMMAS AND STRATEGIES

The above discussion about some of the practical implications of equality of access raises several issues about the distribution and prioritization of health-care services for people affected by HIV and

AIDS, only some of which can be touched on here. Although no one is going to disagree that resources should be targeted to those in need and inefficiencies remedied where they exist, there is a degree of ambivalence in the way central government in the UK has approached this problem. This is reflected in the way diverse elements of managerialism and the market philosophy have been introduced into the NHS. On the one hand practitioners are exhorted to be cost-effective and to achieve 'greater output' with the same or fewer resources: this is the managerial model at work. At the same time they are expected to increase the accessibility of services and provide a more responsive and customized service, pressures which derive from the market model, where the consumer (not the manager) reigns supreme. It is not surprising, then, if nurses feel caught in something of a double-bind by these mixed messages.

The care and social support of people with HIV may need to be shared among a bewildering number of hospital and community providers and agencies, depending on the range of (often unpredictable) conditions and illnesses affecting the individual. With the competing pressures of management and market being brought to bear on the NHS, there appear to be good grounds for arguing that with HIV particular vigilance is required to ensure that people in need are not excluded from vital health care and social support. This cannot be achieved without advocating more and improved resources. There is little point in winning the argument for increased accessibility to testing, care and support if the resources themselves are dwindling or fixed at the status quo. The inevitable result will be an ever-increasing bottleneck at the point of access, more-or-less arbitrary decisions about 'rationing' and probably increased burnout among nursing and other professional staff. So, what role(s) can nurses play in the evolving debate over access?

In addition to their clinical, managerial and broader professional functions, nurses have an important advocacy role. Many of the innovations in HIV prevention and treatment discussed earlier would not have arisen without medical and nursing advocacy. 'Client advocacy' is a term much touted in health care, but does it have any real leverage in a field such as HIV, where clients and carers often advocate quite successfully on their own behalf? Sawyer (1988) sees advocacy as 'the nurse performing a function for a client, which for a number of reasons, he [sic] cannot perform himself'. Carpenter (1992) identifies four reasons why clients may be unable to advocate for themselves:

- illness;
- handicap or level of maturity;

- inhibition due to circumstances (e.g. feeling embarrassed about asking questions);
- lack of knowledge.

We can see how each of these factors might come into play in HIV education and prevention and in the nursing care and management of people with HIV/AIDS. Advocacy is not something that can be left to clients all the time. Not all clients and carers, even the most articulate and resourceful, necessarily have the stamina or determination to ensure that they are consulted in decisions about their needs and wishes, especially by a health-care system which they may perceive as hostile or at best indifferent. The dilemma for nurses lies in reconciling this potential client advocacy role with other roles, such as working cooperatively in a multidisciplinary team. One possible way of approaching this dilemma, as well as tackling the resource management and coordination issue, lies in case management.

There are many definitions of case management and not all of these agree on how a case management programme should be designed, or what practice model is most effective (Kerr and Birk, 1988). However, the most fundamental aspect of case management appears to be 'the designation of one person as a case manager to link each client with needed social and medical services' (Conviser *et al.*, 1991). It thus has an important coordinating function. The three major elements of case management are:

- ensuring access to services;
- continuity of care;
- ultimate responsibility.

Typically, case management is used to link chronically ill populations, such as the mentally ill, the elderly frail or the disabled, with medical and social services. As originally conceived, the case manager is a gatekeeper who determines which primary care providers a client should see. Case managers are also the link person between clients and community-based services; this means that they may have to help to locate or create these services in the first place.

Experience in the United States suggests that case management can also play a vital role in facilitating access to needed medical and social services for people with HIV and AIDS, including those groups who are poorly served by health and welfare systems (Conviser *et al.*, 1991). This is especially important for a group of people subject to rapid changes in their health, and who require rapid access to providers if their needs are to be met. Case managers have also been identified as one of the significant factors in enabling parents and foster families to keep their children with AIDS at home (McGonigel, 1988). From this it can be seen that the role of the case manager may well be vital to the successful mainstreaming of HIV services.

Case managers may be located in acute care settings, health centres (Singh, 1989) and specialist centres, such as drug clinics. Locating case managers at hospitals appears to facilitate client access to care and treatment; such managers are also usually better able to build up a rapport with medical and nursing staff. Locating managers at drug clinics could facilitate the earlier detection and case management of drug users with HIV. An important issue here is flexibility: the appointment of case managers should be determined by individual needs, which will vary. It also goes without saying that service users, user groups and carers should have a say in who or which kind of professional takes on a case management role.

An important aspect of access is the appropriate linkage of people moving from acute care settings to community resources. Occupying a hospital bed and getting the appropriate treatment are by no means the end of the access story. Legislation contained in the NHS and Community Care Act (1990) requires the designation of *care managers* for people with complex care needs. Most people with HIV are likely to fit this description during one or more periods in their life after infection. One study of the coordination of community nursing care of people with HIV/AIDS (Butterworth *et al.*, 1994) indicated that community nurses have to date not been appointed as care managers, even when the greatest input into a patient's care is often community nursing. The study also found a lack of communication between carers in hospital and the community, and an absence of overall coordination. However, the study also reported anecdotal evidence of community nurses taking on this coordinating role, either by default or on the basis of patient choice. It would seem that nurses caring for people with HIV/AIDS in a number of different settings are ideally suited to undertake a management or coordinating role, but that this potential is being tapped only in an ad hoc way.

SUMMARY

A comprehensive range of medical, social and support services should be available and accessible to all people with, or at risk of, HIV. There is still no cure for HIV infection but new developments in prevention and treatment have raised expectations about prognosis and care: these can only lead to increased pressure for access to costly medical investigations and treatments. As HIV infection (in developed countries at least) becomes a more chronic and manageable illness, people with HIV can expect to live relatively more healthy lives. This has additional implications for providing adequate forms of social support and welfare benefits (not discussed here but of equal importance to health care).

Services must be targeted so that limited resources are wisely spent. HIV highlights the uneven, and possibly discriminatory, distribution of health care and other forms of social support. Without special vigilance, particular marginalized groups and individuals affected by HIV who have multiple health-care and social needs are likely to lose out in access to help and support. It is not enough to see accessibility solely in terms of developing a welcoming and user-friendly approach, although this is important. HIV-related initiatives need to be diverse, innovative and often persistent to reach and involve marginalized groups and maintain contact with them. This continues to pose a number of challenges for nursing care. These are likely to continue, however much HIV is integrated into mainstream medical and nursing care.

Top-down pressures to develop a more cost-effective response to HIV prevention and treatment inevitably mean increased competition for scarce resources. Nurses have to date been at the forefront of strategies to increase the accessibility of services to people affected by HIV, especially those who are disadvantaged in society. In addition to their clinical and managerial roles, nurses have an important part to play as client advocates to reduce inequalities of access to care and service provision.

REFERENCES

Arici, C., Finazzi, M. G., Minola, E. *et al.* (1991) Adequacy of case finding and holding of HIV-infected persons. Presentation M.D.4168, 7th International Conference on AIDS, Florence, Italy, 16–21 June.

Bennett, C. and Ferlie, E. (1994) *Managing Crisis and Change in Health Care: the Organizational Response to HIV/AIDS,* Open University Press, Milton Keynes.

Besch, L., Simon, P., Morse, E. *et al.* (1991) Barriers to recruitment and compliance arising from the unique needs of traditionally underserved patient populations. Presentation M.D.4170, 7th International Conference on AIDS, Florence, Italy, 16–21 June.

Bowman, C. A. (1991) The investigation of patients with human immunodeficiency virus infection. *International Journal of STD and AIDS,* **2,** 10–16.

Brettle, R. P., Gore, S. M. and McNeil, A. (1992) Outpatient medical care of injection drug use related HIV. *International Journal of STD and AIDS,* **3,** 96–100.

Butterworth, C. A., Faugier, J. and Brocklehurst, N. (1994) *AIDS and Community Nursing Care: Discharge, Referral Patterns and Coordination*, School of Nursing Studies, University of Manchester.

Carpenter, E. (1992) Advocacy. *Nursing Times Open Learning Supplement*, **88**, 26–7.

Carvell, A. and Hart, G. J. (1990) Help seeking and referrals in a needle exchange: a comprehensive service to injecting drug users. *British Journal of Addiction*, **85**, 235–40.

CDC (1987) Revision of CDC surveillance case definition for acquired immune deficiency syndrome. *Morbidity and Mortality Weekly Report*, **36** (supplement no. 15), 35–115.

CDC (1992) Revised classification system for HIV infection and expanded surveillance case definition for AIDS among adolescents and adults. *Morbidity and Mortality Weekly Report*, **41**, RR17.

Coleman, R., Curtis, D. and Sharpe, M. (1989) The role of the satellite clinic in reaching intravenous drug users at risk from HIV. *Psychiatric Bulletin*, **13**, 165–8.

Concorde Coordinating Committee (1994) Concorde: MRC/ANRS randomised double blind controlled trial of immediate and deferred zidovudine in symptom-free HIV infection. *Lancet*, **343**, 871–81.

Conviser, R., Young, S. R., Grant, C. and Coye, M. J. (1991) A hospital-based case management program of PWAs in New Jersey. *AIDS and Public Policy Journal*, **6**(4), 148–58.

Datt, N. and Feinmann, C. (1990) Providing health care for drug users? *British Journal of Addiction*, **85**, 235–40.

Department of Health (1992a) *The Health of the Nation*, HMSO, London.

Department of Health (1992b) *Guidance on Establishing Additional Sites for HIV Antibody Testing*, PL/CO(92)5, HMSO, London.

Department of Health (1992c) *Guidelines for Offering Voluntary Named HIV Antibody Testing to Women Receiving Ante-natal Care*, PL/CO(92)5, HMSO, London.

Department of Health (1992d) *Children and HIV: Guidance for Local Authorities*, HMSO, London.

Department of Health (1993) *The Health of the Nation Key Area Handbook: HIV/AIDS and Sexual Health*, HMSO, London.

Francis, D. P., Lorien, K., Leven, R. *et al.* (1991) Early intervention: the programme of the future? Initial evaluation. Presentation M.D. 4295, 7th International Conference on AIDS, Florence, Italy, 16–21 June.

Hutchinson, M. and Kurth, A. (1991) 'I need to know I have a choice...': a study of women, HIV and reproductive decision making. *AIDS Patient Care*, February, 17–25.

Irwin, R. (1992) Critical re-evaluation can overcome discrimination: providing equal standards of care for homosexual patients. *Professional Nurse*, April, 435–8.

Katz, M. H., Bindman, A. B., Keane, D. and Chan, A. K. (1991) Early intervention for HIV infection: a gap between theory and practice. Presentation M.D.4169, 7th International Conference on AIDS, Florence, Italy, 16–21 June.

Kerr, M. H. and Birk, J. M. (1988) A client-centred case management model. *Quality Review Bulletin*, **14** (9), 279–83.

Kirk, K. (1992) Descent into darkness. *Gay Times*, June, 27–31.

Lart, R. and Stimson, G. V. (1990) *National Survey of Syringe Exchange Schemes in England*, The Centre for Research on Drugs and Health Behaviour, Charing Cross and Westminster Medical School, London.

Madeley, T. (1987) Having AIDS, in *ABC of AIDS*, (ed M. Adler), British Medical Journal, London, pp. 49–50.

Martin, J. M. and Sacks, H. S. (1990) Do HIV-infected children in foster care have access to clinical trials of new treatments? *AIDS and Public Policy Journal*, **5**, 3–8.

Masur, H. (1990) The changing face of opportunistic infections in the nineties: diagnosis, treatment and monitoring. *AIDS Patient Care*, October, 25–9.

Mays, V. M. and Cochran, S. D. (1991) Physical symptoms and HIV status in US black gay and bisexual men. Presentation M.C.3099, 7th International Conference on AIDS, Florence, Italy, 16–21 June.

McGonigel, M. (1988) *Family Meeting on Paediatric AIDS*, Association for the Care of Children's Health, Washington DC, USA.

McGuiness, R. and Knight, J. (1991) HIV/AIDS prevention work with young people using a mobile unit. Presentation OP-008, 2nd European Conference of Nurses in AIDS Care, Noordwijkerhout, The Netherlands, 19–22 November.

Miller, R., Bor, R., Salt, H. and Murray, D. (1991) Counselling patients with HIV about laboratory tests with predictive values. *AIDS Care*, **3**(2), 159–64.

Mok, J. (1991) HIV infection and children. *British Medical Journal*, **302**, 921–2.

Patton, C. (1990) *Inventing AIDS*, Routledge, London.

Pollak, M. (1992) *AIDS: A Problem for Sociological Research*, Sage, London.

Project Inform (1991) Treatment Strategy, Discussion paper no. 1, San Francisco, USA.

Public Health Laboratory Service (PHLS) Communicable Disease Surveillance Centre (1993) Incidence and prevalence of AIDS and other severe HIV disease in England and Wales for 1992–1997: projections using data to the end of June 1992. *Communicable Disease Report*, **3**, S1–17.

Quaggin, A. (1987) Do doctors consider the risks in research involving children? *Canadian Medical Association Journal*, **136**, 189–91.

Rose, P. and Platzer, H. (1993) Confronting prejudice. *Nursing Times*, **49**(31), 52–4.

Sawyer, J. (1988) On behalf of the patient. *Nursing Times*, **84**(41), 28–30.

Schoenbaum, E. E. and Webber, M. (1991) Underdetection of HIV infection in females seeking care at an inner city emergency room in the Bronx, New York City. Presentation W.C.3093, 7th International Conference on AIDS, Florence, Italy, 16–21 June.

Singh, S. (1989) Liaison with general practice, in *AIDS: Models of Care*, (eds M. Bould and G. Peacock), Kings Fund Centre, London, pp. 35–6.

Stimson, G. V., Aldritt, L., Dolan, K. and Donoghoe, M. (1988) *Injecting Equipment Exchange Schemes: Final Report*, Goldsmiths' College, London.

Strang, J. (1990) The roles of prescribing, in *AIDS and Drug Misuse: the Challenge for Policy and Practice in the 1990s*, (eds J. Strang and G. V. Stimson), Routledge, London, pp. 142–52.

Thomson, A. (1991) Team work to address the issues of HIV/AIDS and drug use in the city. Presentation, 2nd European Conference of Nurses in AIDS Care, Noordwijkerhout, The Netherlands, 19–22 November.

United Kingdom Central Council for Nursing, Midwifery and Health Visiting (UKCC) (1991) *Report on Proposals for the Future of Community Education and Practice*. Post-Registration Education and Practice Project, London.

World Health Organization/European Commission (1993) *Surveillance of AIDS/HIV in Europe*. Quarterly Report no. 39, European Centre for the Epidemiological Monitoring of AIDS, Paris.

Out of sight, out of mind 12

Patrick Coyne and Carmel Clancy

INTRODUCTION

It is well recognized that the data currently available on the prevalence of drug misuse reflect the 'out of sight' nature of the problem. Estimates on drug use in the United Kingdom vary, partly as a result of the wide range and availability of both licit and illicit drugs. That the figures remain hidden should not surprise us, given that illicit drug use is somewhat synonymous with 'covert behaviour'.

The Advisory Council on the Misuse of Drugs (the UK Government's Advisory Body) has repeatedly suggested that there are considerably more than 75 000 injecting drug users in the UK (ACMD, 1989). At present, the only national figures available relating to the nature and extent of drug use are contained within the Home Office Addicts Index and the Department of Health Regional Substance Misuse Databases. Currently there are approximately 20 000 notified drug users, 38% of whom are registered in London (Daniel, *et al.*, 1993). The 'true' figure lies somewhere in the region of five, ten or more times that number. Donoghoe and Stimson (1992) indicated that approximately 10% of London's injecting drug users were HIV seropositive, and approximately 20% of those who injected drugs and who are not in contact with helping agencies may be HIV seropositive.

Nurses of all types, of which there are approximately 500 000 currently practising in Britain, have or will, at some point in their career, come into contact with individuals who have been directly or indirectly affected by problem drug use. Seeking information on the subject, however, shows that most of the literature available is attributed to the work of sociologists, doctors, psychologists and indeed criminologists. The recognition of nurses' work in this 'speciality', and consequently the description of the individual and community being cared for, has gone unnoticed. The lack of visibility is further compounded by the stigma and condemning attitudes which have undoubtedly contributed towards reducing the numbers of people coming forward and identifying themselves. The arrival of HIV/AIDS, along with all the misinformation, fear and prejudice that came with it, has added another important element to this already complex picture. As a consequence, we would suggest that *The Health of the Nation* (Department of Health, 1992b) policies which address HIV and substance misuse, including other target areas such as accidents, cancer, and heart disease, will prove difficult to achieve. Indeed, many of the related targets will be unattainable unless nurses are fully integrated into the plan. In meeting this challenge, nurses will have to become highly visible and vocal to ensure a strategic role for the profession within the public and personal health care arenas.

The Health and Local Authorities, as purchasers of health and social care on behalf of their populations, have a major role in determining the size and shape of their health and social care programmes. The Chief Nursing Officer, Yvonne Moores, has highlighted the essential role of nurses in purchasing health care, and as advisers to purchasers (Kings Fund, 1993). The new culture driving health care provision is based on assessing the health needs of communities, including problematic drug use and concerns about HIV, in order to purchase a high quality and appropriate health care service to meet these needs. It is therefore clear that, if such needs remain hidden, public health is at risk. It must be the responsibility of health care providers (i.e. nurses), in partnership with their colleagues (e.g. other disciplines and voluntary community groups) and the consumers, to inform purchasing intentions.

The importance of informing the purchasing intentions of health authorities, GP fundholders and community care becomes even more relevant in view of the new health care market philosophy. Purchasers, often from non-clinical backgrounds, can only be helped in making sound ethical decisions about the economics of health care if they are informed by all their colleagues in the field (WHO, 1978). Lack of information, understanding and at times empathy, places drug users and the nurses working with them in a marginal position. The challenge of educating our colleagues, the public and the Government on the peculiarities involved in substance misuse remains urgent.

To assist this process, this chapter intends to:

- provide a brief review of the history of substance misuse, and the development of drug and HIV services;

- illuminate nursing works, past and current, which have had a direct impact on the developments of clinical practice, managerial, educational and research work;
- outline what we believe are the future challenges for nursing within this complex and rewarding field.

DRUG MISUSE

The history of drug use or misuse is clouded by the fact that there are a host of words used to describe similar and different phenomena within the field; for example drug misuse, drug use, drug addiction, substance use, substance misuse, drug dependency etc. (Ghodse, 1989). For the purposes of this chapter we will use the term 'problem drug use', meaning the use of chemicals by individuals or groups which lead to harmful impact on the individual and/or the community he/she is part of.

Drugs, including alcohol and tobacco, have been used for centuries by individuals and their communities for a whole host of social, psychological, spiritual and physical reasons (Ghodse and Maxwell, 1990; Kennedy and Faugier, 1989). As a consequence of the harm which may follow the use of drugs, various attempts have been made to place controls on them. One of the first attempts in Britain was the 'Defence of the Realm Act Regulations' in 1916 which made it an offence to possess cocaine and opium (Spear and Mott, 1992). Since then, problem drug use has grown to include the harmful use of a variety of stimulants, hallucinogens and sedatives. In 1967, as a consequence of the second Brain Committee, the Dangerous Drugs Act recommended a system of notification of addicts, special licensing of doctors to prescribe controlled drugs, and the opening of specialist clinics to manage the treatment of drug addicts. Although these new policies undoubtedly assisted many individuals already affected, the ensuing two decades continued to witness an increase in problem drug use. Over that period, the range of drugs available and the diversity of groups using illicit drugs expanded. Problem drug use was not only an issue for individuals and their families, but slowly and insidiously became a problem for society as a whole. It is no longer someone else's concern but has reached in and claimed individuals and communities from all social classes. The advent of HIV and AIDS and the relationship between the virus and problem drug use only served to emphasize this point. This led the ACMD reports of 1988 and 1989 to highlight the threat to public health and seek the re-orientation of drug services from the abstinence model to 'harm minimization' and 'risk reduction'.

SERVICE DEVELOPMENT AND RESPONDING TO NEED

Whilst the 'specialist drug clinics' set up in the late 1960s were responding to the obvious visible need, there was a growing recognition that statutory services could not, and should not, provide all the services for this client group. The non-governmental organizations, now often referred to as the Voluntary and the Independent Sector, many of whom had been set up prior to the establishment of the 'specialist clinics', were in the business of providing complementary services. In the early days, this ranged from self-help groups such as Alcoholics Anonymous (AA) and Narcotics Anonymous (NA), to more crusading efforts from groups such as the Salvation Army.

A significant change for service development was heralded when, in 1982, the ACMD recommended that direct funding from central government should be made available for the development of local drug projects. With hindsight, this Central Funding Initiative, which pump-primed the establishment of local services, allowed services to be in a position to respond to HIV and its spread more rapidly than perhaps other countries. Approximately 250 projects had been set up by 1986 in the UK, including Health Authorities, Voluntary Organizations and Local Authorities (Home Office, 1986). In 1986 and 1987, the initiative allowed for further expansion by 'ring fencing' money specifically for drug services, including extra sums of money for any service addressing HIV prevention as part of its service specifications. This expansion was community-led, with special emphasis on establishing community drug teams (CDTs) and counselling and advisory services. It is interesting to note that a significant proportion of the staff employed in these new services were nurses, who not only had to transfer their skills into this new arena, but also played a leading role in much of the development and health promotion work. Thus non-governmental organizations, such as the Terence Higgins Trust, which sought to involve the Government in the fight against HIV, were being informed by many individuals and groups, including nurses working with the THT drugs advisory group. Gaze (1988a) supported this view by reporting on the voluntary work nurses were actively involved in, determining strategic and direct client care outside of formal statutory frameworks.

A review of service development between 1982 and 1992 was conducted to inform the Working Group for the ACMD report published in 1993 and, not surprisingly, the results confirm the impact of the Central Funding Initiative. Table 12.1 gives details of the development in drug services over that period.

Table 12.1 The growth of drug services 1982–1992

Services	1982		1986		1992	
	Number	% of total	Number	% of total	Number	% of total
Hospital services total	37	100	84	100	89	100
Both in and outpatient	8	22	34	40	60	67
Prescribing	24	65	46	55	71	80
Community services total	20	100	94	100	287	100
Evening/ weekend	6	30	8	9	68	24
Therapeutic groups	4	20	0	0	170	59
Home visits	3	15	4	4	226	79
Detached/ outreach	2	10	1	1	175	61
Skills training	6	30	0	0	no data	no data
Relatives' support	5	25	0	0	no data	no data
Prescribing	–	–	4	4	103	36
Needle exchange	–	–	–	–	214	75
Women's services	–	–	–	–	94	33
After care	–	–	–	–	189	66
Residential services total	25		36		72	

(ACMD, 1993)

DATA AVAILABLE ON THE RELATIONSHIP BETWEEN PROBLEM DRUG USE AND HIV/AIDS

Although services have been developed to meet the challenges of HIV, the impact of the epidemic affecting drug users is difficult to quantify due to the problems previously mentioned in surveying this 'hard to reach' population. However, recent European Surveillance data (AIDS Surveillance in Europe, 1994) indicates that the majority of HIV seropositive people in Italy – 14 120 (66.1%), and Spain – 15 518 (65.8%) have acquired the virus through drug use. In Bangkok and Edinburgh, rapid spread of HIV amongst intravenous drug users has been described, with up to 60% testing positive (ACMD, 1989). In the UK, the number of people known to be HIV seropositive had reached a cumulative total of 22 059 in June 1994, approximately 13% of whom appear to have acquired the virus through drug use (PHLS, 1994). 667 of those individuals who are known to be HIV-1 seropositive have gone on to be diagnosed with AIDS.

It would be impossible to write on problem drug use without at least mentioning, albeit briefly, the numerous reports and government initiatives which have had a particularly important role to play in altering or influencing public health policies on this issue, 'forcing' practitioners to reassess their own role and practices, not only within the treatment and care arenas, but equally within law enforcement, child care, nursing professional development, health, prevention and education.

Although drug policies were on the government's agenda prior to the HIV/AIDS era, arguably their impact on services was minimal. This altered significantly in the mid to late 1980s when document after document was being published on how drug services should be attempting to address the threat to public health of HIV/AIDS. The most significant of these were the Advisory Council on the Misuse of Drugs' reports (1988 and 1989), which re-orientated services towards wider public health issues, emphasizing the need to prevent the spread of HIV. In addition to the public health focus, there were recommendations to include epidemiology and new methods of service delivery such as: outreach, injecting equipment exchanges, greater variety in prescribing treatments and greater involvement of all health and social services who come into contact with individuals or groups affected by problem drug use.

Legislation also had its impact on service development, such as the Children Act (Department of Health, 1992a) which reorientated child care and consequently nurses involved with families towards supporting children within their families rather than removing them. The recent changes in the criminal justice system have sought to increase the options available to the courts, including the possibility of treatment for those found engaging in criminal activity as a result of their problem drug use.

Not only have nurses informed and implemented these policies in providing health care for individuals and communities challenged by substance misuse and HIV/AIDS, they have also being reviewing and making policy on nursing itself. At a time when health and social care is being re-directed into the community, there has been a strategic and unrelenting root-and-branch review of the relevance of nursing to society. In Britain, the *Strategy for Nursing* (Department of Health, 1989) set specific targets for the profession in order to ensure that qualified nurses were not only providing health care, but also leading the efficient and effective provision of this health care. This gave added strength to the developing public health work of nurses in the field of substance misuse. These reviews have recently been enhanced by the updated strategy for nursing (NHS Management Executive, 1993) and the recent review of Mental Health Nursing (Department of Health, 1994).

Most recently, the ACMD (1993) altered the focus of work with problem drug use. The emphasis is now placed on reducing the extent of drug use itself and of injecting, in the hope that this strategy will ultimately contribute to HIV prevention (ACMD, 1993). Following this report, a Central Drugs Co-ordination Unit (CDCU) was set up, with the aim of developing a national drugs strategy. To enhance this work, a Governmental Task Group – the effectiveness review – was established to survey current services, with a view to explore and evaluate how effective they are in helping clients towards a drug free lifestyle and harm minimization.

Nurses need to ensure that policies take into account the need to maintain health gain (Department of Health, 1992b). They must also recognize that new generations of problem drug users, involved with potentially new varieties of drugs and methods of drug use, will require the education and involvement of services that have been developed over the last decade. There can be little doubt that an objective and sensitive evaluation of current policies and services is needed, and nurses must ensure that their successful public health work with clients is clearly visible and subject to evaluation in order to inform and lead this debate.

In general, nursing has a strong history of working with both individuals (Henderson, 1969) and 'the public' (Nightingale, 1992; Zerwekh, 1991), and can be categorized in many ways. The International Congress on Nursing (ICN) suggests four principles of nursing work: the promotion of health, the prevention of illness, the restoring of health and the alleviation of suffering (Department of Health, 1989). We believe nursing work also includes the principles of maintenance of health as well as rehabilitation. For the purposes of examining nursing work in the field of problematic drug use, these principles of nursing practice will be explored, with examples of clinical nursing, management, education and research.

In the light of the history of public health nursing, nurses are well placed to initiate health care responses around HIV related behaviours. Much of their work is about motivating people to improve their health by involving them with helping services. As well as motivating people to consider and attempt improvements in their health behaviours, e.g. safer sex, seeking stable accommodation, resolving legal problems, finding work or collecting their benefits, nurses help clients maintain these improvements to their health and social functioning. When periods of health are challenged by break-ups in relationships, loss of employment, illness or through the death of friends or family, nurses provide support to clients by helping them manage periods of lapse or relapse positively. The work is generally viewed as part of the individual's overall development and maturation, and is highly dependent upon a trusting relationship with both the individual carers and care teams (Egan, 1986). Whilst many in society reject people who use drugs, HIV and AIDS notwithstanding, nurses working in the area of problem drug use have learnt to transform negative feelings and attitudes into a therapeutic neutrality (Chenitz and Krumenaker, 1987). This assists the process of acceptance and respect, and helps to orientate clients towards reality and to manage the potential, or actual, harmful consequences of their behaviours.

Measuring outcomes of nursing work is becoming more possible as quality assurance and resources come into the hands of nurses. Historically, 'success' was viewed by many lay and professional people as abstinence. Nurses working with problem drug users have always viewed, albeit pragmatically, the fact that the client was alive for the next appointment as a 'success', highlighting the high morbidity and mortality associated with drug use. Whilst those outside the field may regard the achievement of abstinence as the only successful outcome, there exists a spectrum of primary and intermediate outcomes which must also be viewed as 'success'. We believe successful outcomes can include :

- engagement of problem drug users into health and social agencies,
- reduction or cessation of the use of 'street drugs' or poly-drug use,
- practising protected penetrative sexual intercourse with casual and regular partners,

- achieving or maintaining employment,
- maintaining positive relations within the family,
- stable accommodation.

Whilst such behaviour changes are being monitored, they are of little value unless nurses and others can provide the on-going care needed to maintain changes, i.e. managing lapses and preventing relapse (Marlatt and Gordon, 1985). In addition, we need to remember that a new generation of problem drug users will enter drug use almost as naively as their predecessors, leaving the question of who will actively encourage the young to get into good health care habits.

PRACTICE

The role of nurses in the area of preventing the epidemic spread of HIV amongst problem drug users is crucial. Examples of nursing practice abound in the field of addiction, concerning promotion, prevention, restoration of health and alleviation of illness. Thus, Staff (1993) describes the work of a community drug team in an area of relatively low HIV prevalence. This group of nurses surveyed their clients for Hepatitis C antibodies and found a high level of prevalence; this worried them because of the suspected similarity with HIV in its transmission process. As a consequence, the nurses were challenged to reflect upon their HIV-risk reduction work, and their research revealed that many of their clients were cleaning their injecting equipment. Although this appeared to reduce the chance of transmitting HIV, the robust Hepatitis C organism remained untouched by such cleaning strategies. From then on, the work of the team with clients incorporated this new feature by enhancing the risk reduction work so that it now took into account the risk of Hepatitis C transmission, i.e. only unshared equipment should be used, and individual injecting equipment should be cleaned separately.

The use of 'labels' to empower clients has been harnessed to offer problem drug users health education about HIV. Rather than using the labels 'AIDS Interview' or indeed 'Counselling and Testing', Coyne, Lambert and Boyjoonauth (1993) developed a 'Health Interview', offering clients of substance misuse services a brief health-focused intervention, aimed at managing stress and promoting health in the area of substance use and sexual behaviour. Whilst clients seek help to manage problematic drug use, this intervention serves to highlight their personal resource strengths, and to confirm and affirm successful self-help strategies.

Health promotion can be enhanced by the use of counselling theory. Robinson (1989) concluded that there was significant evidence for counselling to be recognized as a powerful helping intervention. This may seem very difficult, e.g. when it comes to promoting healthy pregnancy in cases where the mother may or may not be seropositive and the child is at risk. However, Roth and Brierly (1989) highlighted many of the issues associated with making this experience a constructive health encounter for the mother, child and family: for this to happen, the nurse needs to ensure good communication and liaison skills between carers and the mother. Sophisticated communication is particularly vital if the mother is dependent on drugs, where liaison with specialists in the area of substance misuse is required. Wason, a clinical liaison nurse specialist, has developed a network of services meeting this criteria (Wason and Dale, 1991).

For drug users who are HIV seropositive, there is evidence that health is more likely to be restored and maintained when lifestyles are immuno-supportive, i.e. where harm due to stress is minimized, and health is promoted. Nurses are central to this. A senior nurse's work in the drop-in clinic in Rathbone Place, London, shows how chaotic drug users can be engaged into health services which offer substitution drug programmes, detoxification, rehabilitation, or allow them to receive long term methadone maintenance and its associated supportive counselling, education, and supply of condoms (Ward *et al.*, 1992). A further example of this type of work is demonstrated by the availability of Well-Women services to female drug users, allowing them to have family planning information, smears and breast screening, a service offered by many community drug and outreach teams (Jones, 1994; Riverside Health Promotions, 1992).

The Griffin Project, which is a nursing centre for active drug users who are HIV seropositive and symptomatic, has been established in London (Turning Point, 1991). It aims to provide nursing care for those seriously affected by HIV and with a history of substance use. The nursing practices include post acute care, convalescent care, respite care and terminal care. For those in the community who are problem drug users and HIV seropositive, the Healthy Options Team in Bloomsbury included a nurse whose role was to offer assistance with rehabilitation programmes and enable clients to maximize their potential in a variety of ways, e.g. by helping them to develop support networks so that they can lead as independent a life as possible (Elward, 1993).

MANAGEMENT

Nurses have a major role in the development of health services, particularly their conceptual design and implementation (Black and

Boyjoonauth, 1985; Fraser, 1994). Since the development of the NHS Drug Advisory Services (DAS/HAS) in 1986, nursing has been selected as a key discipline essential for the management and provision of health and social care in this field, making nurses highly influential in the development and improvement of substance misuse services. Thus, in 1991, the DAS recommended to South West Durham during a visit that the Community Addictions Advisory Service should seek the advice and support of the clinical nurse specialist (HIV/AIDS) in the managerial development of a community based syringe exchange scheme, thereby acknowledging the role of a clinical nurse specialist as a valuable managerial resource.

Nurses have been involved with identifying resources to promote health. During the first European Drug Prevention Week in 1992 (Davidson, 1993), they were specifically involved in targeting young people about problem drug use. The 'Action for Sound Health' initiative of East Surrey Health Promotion Unit co-ordinated a multi-agency input to this project. Based on the assumption that promoting health amongst young people requires pertinent and attractively presented issues, the project attended young people's social venues. It incorporated information quizzes and other activities into the fun and enjoyment of the social occasions. The evaluation of the work showed this approach to be a most successful way of reaching a young audience in an informal social context. This contradicts the fear-based approaches of many health projects, and focuses on health as pleasure, enjoyment and the satisfactory use of one's potential.

Partners are often the ones who provide most care for those affected by HIV illness. A relatively recent phenomenon on the British HIV scene is the provision of care by the female partners of HIV seropositive men. Thurton (1992) describes some of the issues associated with managing a community nursing response to such families. Acting as a major support to partners, many of whom may themselves be seropositive, highlights yet another role for community nurses working with seropositive families, especially where drug use is involved. The need to design management strategies to ensure that nurses are supported and supervised in order to remain in this work, represents a major responsibility for managers (Butterworth and Faugier, 1992).

The availability of suitable accommodation is a challenging aspect of care, especially at a time of great homelessness. Chamberlin (1989) reviewed a number of housing models for those affected by HIV, and made recommendations for those managing the development of housing projects. They noted that drug users lacked many of the social structures that provide the background for gay support organizations, and pointed to the need to develop housing for those on the fringes of society due to drug use and illegal activity. Faced with the challenge of HIV, ROMA (a residential rehabilitation service for drug users being prescribed medication) developed a nursing service aimed at reducing the health needs of problem drug users who may be either seropositive or at high risk of becoming so. At the same time, this service retained the rehabilitation elements of its work (Byrne, 1993). They managed this change of aims and objectives, and the incorporation of nursing, in order to offer a challenging and innovative service to clients.

EDUCATION

Within the areas of HIV and problem drug use, education on issues related to drug and sexual practices has made enormous strides. This has arguably taken several forms, including the education of nurses themselves and the provision of health education for individuals and the wider community. The ACMD (1982) recommended an increased provision of pre- and post-qualification education about problem drug use for professional staff. These courses were set up with the help of a variety of funding, including the *Central Funding Initiative 1983–1989* (Home Office, 1988). The courses incorporated education about HIV; thus, Manchester's English National Board course on drugs and alcohol included the *ENB 943 – Care and Management of people with HIV and AIDS*. The need to change nursing education to take on board both the issues of problem drug use and HIV has led to dramatic changes.

In the early days of the epidemic, it became apparent that a clear and reflective awareness of infection control and universal precautions was a fundamental issue for the development of a humanitarian and safe response for this client group (Pratt, 1988). Isolation and the use of 'space suits' to provide nursing care are generally part of history. Sadler (1987) advocated the education of the nurse for the provision not only of information about HIV and its transmission, but also of the means by which this information can be turned into actual practice. Gaze (1988b) supported this view, stating that the atmosphere required to promote health needs to be positive and constructive, in contrast to the uninformed and fearful practice prevalent during the early days of the epidemic.

Nurses have done much of the liaison work with acute and primary medical services to help HIV-positive problem drug users receive out-patient and in-patient medical care. The Department of Health's video series on *Nursing and AIDS* includes a specific video and booklet on drug misuse (Department of Health, 1991; Coyne, Wilson and Jackesley,

1991). This health education package is a partnership between problem drug users and nurses, explaining how substance misuse services work, and how they could function in partnership with other health and social services to provide a health care service to clients who use drugs, have HIV concerns, and require nursing care.

RESEARCH

Nursing has often been described as being both an art and a science. The former has always been well recognized within and outside the profession, while the latter suffered from being under-valued, under-resourced and often undermined. Against this backdrop, particularly over the past four decades, nurses have endeavoured to redress the balance, and their tenacity is reflected in the number of nurses now involved in the area of research, within which, the subjects of HIV and problem drug use, although not necessarily obvious, are abundant.

An example has been identified with the work of Coyne, Meadows, Catalan and Wells (1991). In order to target health education toward the prevention of transmission of HIV in individuals and populations, they surveyed a cohort of drug service attendees in an area of relatively high HIV seroprevalence to identify their awareness and attitudes with regard to HIV and health behaviours. Whilst most were generally aware of risk, and many showed signs of changes in health behaviours, e.g. greater use of condoms with casual partners than with regular partners; the changes were not adequate to protect themselves or others. The most commonly identified thoughts and feelings about not using condoms were associated with the possibility of creating problems within important sexual relationships. They discovered as a result of this research that health care need goes well beyond providing information and materials, with clients needing the opportunity to discuss and overcome on-going difficulties with health behaviour changes in a confidential and trusting relationship.

Nurses, who have been involved in conducting in depth surveys on problem drug users, their attitudes and sexual behaviours, suggest that not only do drug users contradict the conventional wisdom that problem opiate users have 'no sex lives', but that many put themselves at high risk of damage to their health as a result of their active sexual choices. The complexity of these behaviours is highlighted by the paradox of most injecting drug users being aware of the possibility that they may be seropositive and at the same time not consciously believing that they are putting their partners at serious risk (Klee, Faugier, Hayes, Boulton and Morris, 1990). This kind of research has been essential in informing practice in the field of health promotion and health maintenance.

Within the last decade nurses' work in the area of substance misuse has highlighted and affirmed the role of nurses as leaders in health care provision. The onset of graduate training, research, publications, including books like this, and policy review, reveal how nurses are beginning to take their long awaited position within the scientific community. As a consequence, their views and opinions are observed with greater respect.

For the future, policy changes need to be critically evaluated by nurses. The recent change towards public health from individual-focused health, emphasizes this, in possibly precluding the individual from receiving the respect, acceptance and empathy that individuals require from nurses when they have health concerns. This is particularly pertinent in the area of problem drug use when drawing on our experience of liberal prescribing of methadone to intravenous drug users, from the mid-1980s. This was arguably implemented as a 'social control measure' against the spread of HIV to the general public, rather than considering the personal health needs of the individual problem drug user.

Remaining 'out of sight' of other disciplines, including managers and policy makers, prevents a true and complete picture of our clients being perceived, and also prevents the promotion of nursing theory at the predictive and prescriptive levels (Dickoff, James and Wiedenbach, 1968). A strategic development of nursing literature and research is urgently required (Hennessy and Cooper, 1994) and we would argue specifically within substance misuse.

The existence of specialist drug and HIV services, although needed, is not enough. Whilst progress has been made, in liaison with generic health services, the dilemma remains about how to enhance mainstream primary, secondary and tertiary care for people using drugs. There is also a strong argument, that with supportive education and training, primary care teams are better placed to manage uncomplicated problematic drug use and HIV, not to mention their role in prevention and early detection. Nurses, as a discipline, are potentially the most appropriate candidates to take on this developmental work, based on their breadth of education and experiences in a variety of health care settings.

Some of the most important challenges facing nurses in the field of substance misuse and HIV are the concepts of the 'internal market', 'needs assessment' and 'competition'. These provide both opportunities and threats to the provision of quality health care. Nurses need to be vigilant in safeguarding the rights of their client group, ensuring that they have 'open access' to drug services. One of the most important opportunities from the changes is the involvement of problem drug users in the development of services. The challenge for nurses is to ensure that the needs of their clients are addressed through improved standard setting and multidisciplinary audit. Whilst progress has been made with user groups, exciting opportunities remain.

Nurses, who are singularly the most employed discipline within the field of substance misuse, and yet rarely describe their work have a responsibility to change this situation for the good of the nation's health. This problem is further compounded by the camouflage of nursing work under the guise of 'drug worker'. Whilst we wholly agree that health care delivery is about skill sharing, multidisciplinary and multiagency cooperation (Coyne and Dhanani, 1993), this is only possible if the individual disciplines with their different histories, knowledge bases, experiences and practices, are clear about their theory and practice. To offer holistic care, rigorous reflection upon the whole and the parts of the whole is required.

Part of the responsibility for increasing nurses' confidence in recording and publishing their work lies within the domain of nurse education. Due to the multiple roles of nurses within the field of substance misuse and HIV, there is a striking need to enhance not only their basic education but particularly their post-basic education as clinical nurse specialists. Leiker (1989) describes the role of the 'addictions nurse specialist' as applying nursing theory; acting as a role model and teacher to the client and colleagues; assessing, devising, and evaluating treatment plans and liaising with other departments and professionals. Critical to this role development, is active membership of professional organizations. Such membership facilitates sharing of good practice and the development of nursing knowledge. The specialism of addictions is often a stigmatized and difficult area in which to work, the field needs articulate, powerful and knowledgeable ambassadors.

The need to enhance and maintain caring attitudes and services, in an increasingly indifferent society, to this challenging and vulnerable group has never been more imperative.

REFERENCES

Advisory Council on the Misuse of Drugs (1982) *Treatment and Rehabilitation.* HMSO, London.
Advisory Council on the Misuse of Drugs (1988) *AIDS and Drug Misuse: Part 1.* HMSO, London.

Advisory Council on the Misuse of Drug (1989) *AIDS and Drug Misuse: Part 2.* HMSO, London.

Advisory Council on the Misuse of Drugs (1993) *AIDS and Drug Misuse.* HMSO, London.

AIDS Surveillance in Europe (1994) Quarterly Report No 41, 31 March. European Centre for the Epidemiological Monitoring of AIDS, Saint-Maurice.

Black, E. and Boyjoonauth, R. (1985) Shaping the future pattern of community nursing services (mental health). *Nursing Practice,* **1,** 43–50.

Butterworth, T. and Faugier, J. (eds.) (1992) *Clinical Supervision and Mentorship in Nursing.* Chapman & Hall, London.

Byrne, G. (1993) *Crisis Intervention and Drug Maintenance in Residential Settings.* Association of Nurses in Substance Abuse (ANSA): 9th National Conference, Chester, UK.

Chamberlin, R. (1989) Homeless Drug Users with HIV Infection, in *Caring for People with AIDS in the Community: Nursing Fellowships,* a summary of reports (Department of Health). HMSO, London.

Chenitz, W.C. and Krumenaker, C. (1987) The Nurse in a Methadone Maintenance Clinic: Revisited. *Journal of Psychosocial Nursing,* **25**(11), 13–17.

Coyne, P.F., Meadows, J., Catalan, P. and Wells, B. (1991) *A Study of the Use of Condoms by Drug Dependency Clinic Attenders to Enable the Provision of Accurately Directed HIV Health Care Work.* International Conference on AIDS/II STD World Congress, Florence, Italy.

Coyne, P., Wilson, D. and Jackesley, H. (1991) *Nursing and AIDS: Drug Misuse.* HMSO, London.

Coyne, P.F., Lambert, L. and Boyjoonauth, R. (1993) *Public Health – Developing an Interview for Health: Motivational Health Promotion Interview on HIV Health Risk Reduction.* Association of Nurses in Substance Abuse (ANSA). 9th National Conference; Chester, UK.

Coyne, P. and Dhanani, G. (1993) Working with HIV Illness. *Drug Link,* Jan/Feb, 14–15.

Daniel, P., Brown, A., Jones, M. and Morgan, D. (1993) *Problem Drug Use by Services in Greater London: A Collaborative Report by Regional Drug Misuse Databases.* St George's Medical School, London.

Davidson, L. (1993) in *European Drug Prevention Week: Evaluation Report* (C. Clancy), SW Thames Regional Drug and Alcohol Team, St George's Hospital Medical School, London.

Department of Health (1989) *A Strategy for Nursing.* HMSO, London.

Department of Health (1991) *Nursing and AIDS: Drug Misuse* (Video). HMSO, London.

Department of Health (1992a) *The Children Act: An Introductory Guide for the NHS.* HMSO, London.

Department of Health (1992b) *The Health of the Nation.* HMSO, London.

Department of Health (1994) *Working in Partnership: A Review of Mental Health Nursing.* HMSO, London.

Dickoff, J.J., James, P.A. and Wiedenbach, E. (1968) Theory in a practice discipline 1: practice-orientated discipline. *Nursing Research,* **17,** 415–35.

Donoghoe, M. and Stimson, G.V. (1992) *HIV prevalence highest in London injecting drug users with no treatment or previous testing history.* Abstract number PUC8062. VIII International Conference on AIDS, Amsterdam.

Drug Advisory Service (DAS) (1991) *Report by the NHS Advisory Service on Services for Problem Drug Users in the South West Durham Health District.* National Health Service Health Advisory Services, London.

Egan, G. (1986) *The Skilled Helper: A Systematic Approach to Effective Helping.* 3rd edn, Brooks/Cole, California.

Elward, J. (1993) *Community based terminal care for drug users with HIV disease.* Association of Nurses in Substance Abuse: ninth national conference; Chester; UK.

Fraser, H. (1994) *Towards a District Health Strategy for Substance Misuse.* Department of Public Health Medicine, Merton and Sutton Health Authority, London.

Gaze, H. (1988a) AIDS: a growth industry. *Nursing Times,* **84**(21), 16–17.

Gaze, H. (1988b) Has a dream come true? *Nursing Times,* **84**(41), 16–17.

Ghodse, H. (1989) *Drugs and Addictive Behaviour: A Guide to Treatment.* Blackwell, Oxford.

Ghodse, H. and Maxwell, D. (1990) *Substance Dependency: An Introduction for the Caring Professions.* Macmillan, London.

Henderson, V. (1969) *Basic principles of nursing care.* International Council of Nurses, Geneva.

Hennessy, D. and Cooper, S. (1994) Co-ordinated Strategy. *Nursing Times,* **90**(28), 42–3.

Home Office (1986) *Tackling Drug Misuse: A Summary of the Government's Strategy.* 2nd edn. HMSO, London.

Home Office (1988) *Tackling Drug Misuse: A Summary of the Government's Strategy.* 3rd edn. HMSO, London.

Jones, G. (1994) Women's Drop-In: Drugs and AIDS Counselling and Advisory Service (DACAS). Substance Misuse Bulletin, April, 6, p.8. SW Thames Regional Drug and Alcohol Team, London.

Kennedy, J. and Faugier, J. (1989) *Drug and alcohol dependency nursing.* Heinemann, Oxford.

Kings Fund (1993) *The professional nursing contribution to purchasing.* NHSME Nursing Directorate, London.

Klee, H., Faugier, J., Hayes, C. *et al.* (1990) Sexual partners of injecting drug users: the risk of HIV infection. *British Journal of Addiction,* **85**, 413–18.

Leiker, T.L. (1989) The role of the addictions nurse specialist in a general hospital setting. *Nurses Clinics of North America,* **24**(1), 137–49.

Marlatt, G.A. and Gordon, J.R. (1985) *Relapse Prevention: Maintenance Strategies in the Treatment of Addictive Behaviors.* Guilford Press, New York.

NHS Management Executive (1993) *A Vision for the Future: The Nursing, Midwifery and Health Visiting Contribution to Health and Health Care.* Department of Health, London.

Nightingale, F. (1992) *Notes on Nursing.* Commemorative edition. Lippincott, Philadelphia.

Pratt, R.J. (1988) *AIDS: A Strategy for Nursing Care,* 2nd edn. Edward Arnold, London.

Public Health Laboratory Service (1994) *AIDS and HIV Infection in the UK*. Monthly report 15 July, **4**(28), 131–2.

Riverside Health Promotions (1992) *Rapid assessment service for drug users*. HIV Agenda: newsletter for primary carers in Riverside. RHP, London.

Robinson, D. (1989) Drug use, HIV infection and change in risk behaviour, in *Caring for people with AIDS in the community: nursing fellowships*, a summary of reports (Department of Health). HMSO, London.

Roth, C. and Brierley, J. (1989) HIV and pregnancy. *Nursing Times*, **85**(6), 73–4.

Sadler, C. (1987) Who's at risk? *Nursing Times*, **87**(18), 27–31.

Spear, H.B. and Mott, J. (1992) in *Crack and Cocaine in England and Wales: Research and Planning Unit Paper 70* (ed. J. Mott). Home Office, London.

Staff, A. (1993) *Has pragmatic euphoria undermined the gospel of good health?* Association of nurses in substance abuse: ninth national conference; Chester, UK.

Thurton, P. (1992) Families and HIV: united we stand. *Nursing Times*, **88**(5), 29–31.

Turning Point (1991) *Turning Point Griffin Project: Continuing Care Unit*. Turning Point, London.

Ward, J., Dark, S., Hall, W. and Mattick, R. (1992) Methadone maintenance and the human immunodeficiency virus: current issues in treatment and research. *British Journal of Addiction*, **87**, 447–53.

Wason, G. and Dale, A. (1991) *Report of liaison nurse specialist drug services for women, ethnic and other minorities groups*. Riverside Substance Misuse Service, London.

Wells, R. (1985) Express train to death. *Nursing Mirror*, **160**(7), 16–18.

World Health Organisation (1978) *Primary Health Care*. Report of the international conference on primary health care, Alma-Ata, USSR. WHO, Geneva.

Zerwekh, J.V. (1991) Public health nursing legacy: a historical practical wisdom. *Nursing and Health Care*, **13**(2), 84–91.

FURTHER READING

Coyne, P.F., Donoghoe, M., Hunter, G. and Stimson, G. (1992) *Condom Usage by London Injecting Drug Users (IDUs) in 1990 and 1991*. VIII International Conference/II STD World Congress, Amsterdam, Holland.

Health Education Authority (1993) *Health of the Nation*. AIDS Dialogue, **18**, 13.

Higgins, D.L., Galavotti, C., O'Reilly, K.R. *et al.* (1991) Evidence for the effects of HIV antibody counselling and testing on risk behaviours. *Journal of the American Medical Association*, **266**(17), 2419–29.

Kelly, S. (1992) Lowering the odds. *Nursing Times*, **88**(9), 42–3.

Kelly, S. (1992) *A new day, a new policy, a new cutback...a new approach – addiction prevention in primary care*. Association of nurses in substance abuse: ninth national conferene; Chester, UK.

Seymour, J. (1991) Primary aid. *Nursing Times*, **87**(24), 19.

Sims, R. (1988) Practical nursing aspects. *Nursing Standard*, August 20, 26–7.

Trevelyan, J. (1988) Climate of fear: three projects are being set up for AIDS patients. *Nursing Times*, **84**(18), 27–31.

Marrying mind and matter

13

Stephen Firn

INTRODUCTION

A large body of literature now exists which associates HIV infection and AIDS with a wide variety of mental health problems. First, this includes people who have not been infected with HIV but have excessive concerns about acquiring the virus, or falsely believe or assert that they have been infected. Secondly, a number of psychosocial conditions have been identified, such as anxiety states and mood disturbances, as a reaction to the changes and losses associated with living with the virus. Thirdly, HIV has been shown to cause a number of neuropsychiatric disorders. These include opportunistic infections and tumours affecting the brain as a result of immunosuppression, and the primary effects of HIV infecting the central nervous system causing a condition known as HIV-associated dementia. Finally, a minority of people with HIV experience psychotic illnesses such as hypomania and severe depression.

Conflicting accounts have been published regarding both the prevalence and the aetiology of many of the mental health problems in HIV disease. It is not possible in this chapter to do justice to the depth and complexity of this literature. Comprehensive reviews are available elsewhere (Everall and Lantos, 1991; Maj, 1990a). However, the main areas of agreement and the key points of debate about mental health problems in HIV disease will be summarized and an attempt made to show the relevance of these issues to nursing care. Care examples will be used to illustrate the challenges that mental health problems can present to the effective nursing care and management of people affected by HIV, to highlight instances of good nursing practice and offer advice and possible solutions.

This chapter is intended to be of value to both psychiatric and general nurses, since the multifaceted nature of HIV disease means that nurses caring for people with the virus frequently find themselves assessing and responding to both physical and mental health needs. Often it is difficult, if not impossible, to separate the two. In this sense, the care of HIV-infected people demands a truly holistic approach, and all nurses working in this field should strive to develop an awareness of the mental health concerns and at least feel able to ascertain when referral to a specialist may be necessary.

MENTAL HEALTH PROBLEMS AFFECTING PEOPLE NOT KNOWN TO BE INFECTED WITH HIV

DISPROPORTIONATE FEARS OF INFECTION

The ways in which HIV and AIDS have encapsulated and become the focus for intense societal fears, prejudices and concerns has been well documented (Aggleton and Homans, 1988). In recent years more media attention has been devoted to AIDS than to any other public health concern: warnings about the dangers of HIV infection have appeared in advertisements on television, in magazines, on billboards and even on leaflets sent to every home in the UK. At the height of such campaigns many individuals came forward for HIV antibody testing, but the majority were people at minimal or no risk of infection who were disproportionately concerned about being infected (Lewin and Williams, 1988). Most people with such concerns are reassured by interventions such as skilled counselling, the provision of factual information and a negative test result. However, a minority are not, and remain persistently worried and anxious that they are at great risk of becoming infected through everyday activities. This may lead to the development of acute anxiety and even panic attacks, particularly when they find themselves in situations which they fear will place them at risk of infection. In addition, they may develop obsessive rituals such as repeated handwashing and checking of objects for traces of blood or other body fluids (Mathews, 1988).

Others may be excessively fearful that they have already been infected, despite repeated negative test results, and may develop anxiety-based physical symptoms such as tremors, sweating, diarrhoea and loss of appetite. These symptoms are similar to those that can occur in HIV disease and are therefore often interpreted as confirmation of infection. Further features may include repeated bodily checking for signs of HIV disease, such as Kaposi's sarcoma lesions.

Davey and Green (1991) suggested that excessive concerns about AIDS are a 'new face for an old problem'. That is, the symptomatology is very similar to that observed in other hypochondriacal conditions. However, they observe that one additional feature seems to be a fear of infecting loved ones, and this can create additional anxiety and guilt.

People with disproportionate fears about AIDS are often referred to as 'the worried well', but it should be recognized that up to 50% of people with such fears may experience suicidal ideas (Miller *et al.* 1988). The term is also a misnomer if the symptoms interfere to a significant degree with a person's functioning, lead to actual self-harm, and cause great distress to the individuals affected and their loved ones. For example, our team was referred a 55-year-old gentleman who reported that his fears of infection stemmed from stepping on a mark on the pavement that he believed could have been dried blood. No other risk activities were identified. Nevertheless, to try and allay his anxiety he soaked his body in household disinfectant up to ten times a day, and as a result his skin was extremely sore and peeling from his neck downwards. He had taken to wearing gloves to avoid having to touch other people, and this included his family, whom he was terrified of infecting. Not surprisingly, his relationships with other family members were in crisis. He ran his own business and this was in financial trouble because he felt extremely uncomfortable meeting business contacts, owing to his anxiety about contagion and embarrassment about smelling of disinfectant.

Whenever a person's persistent concerns about AIDS are affecting their physical or mental health, or impinging upon their social and personal lives, referral to a mental health professional should be suggested. The aim of such referrals is to assess the extent and possible causes of the concerns, to help patients gain an understanding of the reasons for their anxiety, and to identify techniques for eliminating their symptoms.

ASSESSMENT

A number of predisposing factors have been identified as being linked to the development of HIV-related concerns among the 'worried well' (Davey and Green, 1991; Flaskerud, 1992). The assessment should therefore include consideration of the following factors, which may indicate the source of the concerns and help focus interventions:

- a consideration of any recent stressors or losses in the person's life;
- an assessment for signs of an underlying depressive illness;

- guilt feelings relating to some past behaviour, particularly in relation to a sexual relationship or activity which they did not approve of, or believed others close to them would not approve of either;
- over-concern about other diseases in the past, suggesting that HIV had become the focus for long-standing worries about their health;
- death or the development of serious illness in a close friend or relative in the 6 months prior to the onset of symptoms.

It is important to be as factual as possible and not seek to reassure in the hope that this will relieve the person's anxiety. The giving of reassurance to people with chronic anxiety only serves to increase it (King, 1993). People with excessive fears of infection often want to know exactly how long the virus can survive outside the body, and exactly how much of each body fluid is required to transmit the virus. This is frequently within the context of some imagined scenario, such as drinking from a cup which is somehow tainted with a minute speck of blood from the mouth of a previous user. It should be stated that the risk of infection through such sources is minuscule but cannot be exactly quantified. The patient must then draw his or her own conclusions.

INTERVENTIONS

The first step in assisting people come to terms with their anxieties is to help them to reinterpret their symptoms as being due to a fear of AIDS rather than due to AIDS itself. Flaskerud (1992) reports that simple explanations about the functioning of the autonomic nervous system, along with the skilled use of cognitive–behavioural techniques, has enabled patients to recognize bodily symptoms as physiological expressions of anxiety, rather than symptoms of HIV disease. In addition, cognitive techniques can assist the person to reframe the mental health problem within the context of other stresses and predisposing factors in their life. These interventions can help infected individuals understand the reasons why they are experiencing such anxiety, and thereby begin to reassert control.

Mathews (1988) described the benefits of teaching anxiety-reducing techniques such as deep muscle relaxation and controlled breathing, which can be practised and utilized during gradual exposure to self-identified anxiety-provoking situations or activities. These may include reading AIDS-related literature, or drinking from a cup in a café. Mathews also reported that the use of rational–emotive therapy (RET) had been successful in helping a person with a fear of AIDS replace negative, anxiety-provoking thoughts with positive ones. This approach may be particularly useful with individuals who feel guilty about some past act or behaviour, and have recurrent thoughts about being punished for their 'sins'.

OTHER MENTAL HEALTH PROBLEMS IN PATIENTS NOT HIV POSITIVE

A number of case reports have been made concerning people who present to mental health services with false claims of being HIV positive or having AIDS (McDonald and Wafer, 1989). It has been suggested that this is a contemporary expression of the Munchausen syndrome (Asher, 1951), in which people seek medical help for fictitious illnesses. Certainly, the topical and emotive nature of the syndrome provides an appropriate background to the dramatic and acute presentation which is a feature of the Munchausen syndrome.

A 35-year-old man was referred via casualty after having his stomach pumped following an overdose of analgesics. He claimed his partner had recently died of an AIDS-related illness and that he himself was HIV positive. He remained under constant supervision for the next fortnight, and appeared to be experiencing an acute grief reaction to his partner's death and an adjustment reaction to his own diagnosis. He again attempted self-harm by overdose. However, we were unable to contact his GP, the unit where he said he was tested, or any relatives, as the numbers he gave us were never answered. He agreed to a HIV antibody test, which was negative. We subsequently discovered that he had a 10-year history of presenting with acute grief reactions (although not previously AIDS related) across many hospitals. Unfortunately, upon being told this he left the hospital and did not return, and so we were unable to assess or treat any underlying mental health problem.

Such instances, although relatively rare, demonstrate the importance of always obtaining written confirmation of a person's HIV diagnosis and, if this is not possible, conducting an antibody test. This is now standard practice in many HIV units. Should this prove negative, an antigen test may be considered. The need for this is seemingly reinforced by the occasional reports of people with delusional beliefs that they have AIDS, and of people claiming to be infected with the aim of social or financial gain (King, 1993).

PSYCHOSOCIAL CONCERNS AFFECTING PEOPLE WITH HIV

The most common mental health problems experienced by people with HIV are of a psychosocial nature, that is, they are related to the many psychological and social stresses and losses which can arise as a result of

HIV infection, and they fit into the main categories of adjustment disorders, anxiety disorders and depressive conditions (Catalan, 1993).

A number of factors have been suggested as having particular significance in HIV disease and contributing to the development of psychosocial conditions. These include the problems caused by living with the uncertainty surrounding the progression of HIV disease, coupled with the knowledge that it is a potentially fatal condition. In addition, the stigma and prejudice which continue to surround the virus mean that many people find that support and understanding from loved ones or significant others is not forthcoming. This can have very damaging effects on interpersonal relationships, sexual expression and employment, and often leads to feelings of alienation and rejection, along with possible loss of income and status (King, 1989; Korniewicz *et al.*, 1990; Burnard, 1993). Other authors have pointed out that, in western societies, those primarily affected up to the present time have been people whose lifestyles were stigmatized before the advent of HIV, such as gay men and drug users. These groups may find it particularly difficult to reveal their diagnosis, since it may also entail revealing details of their lifestyle which they had chosen not to disclose in the past. Finally, compared to other life-threatening illnesses, the majority of people affected by HIV are relatively young and may find it particularly hard to cope with debilitating and life-threatening illness (Miller and Riccio, 1990; King, 1990).

Estimates of the number of people experiencing psychosocial problems vary greatly. However, while recognizing that many people will encounter periods and situations when they have great difficulty coping with living with the virus, it should be emphasized that most individuals cope well most of the time. People with HIV and AIDS do not automatically become emotional cripples. To illustrate this point, a study of 192 outpatients with HIV or AIDS found that while 31% had significant psychiatric problems, this level of psychological distress is comparable to that found in studies of people in general medical wards. The author concluded that, overall, the people in this study had adapted well to their diagnosis. In addition, almost half had experienced the symptoms before knowing they were infected, and this suggests that HIV was associated with a recurrence of previous mental health problems rather than being the sole cause of new ones (King, 1989). These findings are supported by Gala *et al.* (1993), who conducted a controlled study comparing 259 asymptomatic seropositive people with 159 who were seronegative. They found that overall levels of current or previous psychiatric disturbance did not differ significantly between HIV-positive or HIV-negative subjects, and that they were similar to those found in other life-threatening conditions. Family problems during childhood and a previous history of emotional disturbance before HIV testing correlated with psychiatric morbidity, and the authors suggest that among asymptomatic individuals these factors are more significant than HIV disease itself. The authors also reported that injecting drug users had significantly higher levels of both past and current psychiatric morbidity than gay men or heterosexuals in the study, and that this was regardless of their HIV status. This suggests that past and current lifestyle may also be a more significant risk factor for psychological distress than HIV infection alone.

Although in many ways these findings are encouraging, since they suggest that most people adapt well to living with the virus, it is also important to remember that some do experience significant psychological distress, often related to particular events during the disease process. A survey of care providers throughout Europe (Catalan, 1993) found that the specific stages which were most commonly associated with psychological distress were, in decreasing order:

- following the development of symptoms;
- after an AIDS diagnosis;
- after HIV diagnosis;
- in response to a decline in laboratory indicators;
- during terminal care stages;
- when prophylaxis is introduced.

Those who appear to be most at risk are:

- people with a previous history of a mental health problem, including substance misuse;
- people with low self-esteem;
- those who say they have few social supports;
- people who have experienced repeated losses to AIDS among their social circle.

(Korniewicz *et al.*, 1990; Miller and Riccio, 1990; King, 1993).

It is important for nurses to be aware of this information, since it can help prevent the onset of problems by anticipating need and can also enable nurses to identify what care and interventions may be required. It is therefore imperative that nurses conduct a detailed mental health assessment, which should include the following areas (Flaskerud, 1992):

Previous psychiatric history HIV-infected people with a previous history of seeking professional help for a mental health problem, including substance misuse, are more vulnerable to a recurrence or exacerbation of psychological distress. They may therefore benefit from being offered increased psychological support, particularly during the stressful periods listed above.

Previous losses to HIV and AIDS People who have experienced repeated losses to AIDS find it more difficult to cope with the effects of their own illness. This may indicate the need for increased psychological support and planning of coping strategies in the event of future changes and losses.

Current psychological and social concerns Assess whether the patient is currently experiencing any fears or concerns and, if so, which are the most worrying. It may be helpful for the nurse to try to help the patient identify those which can be dealt with there and then, such as lack of information about treatment or illness, or concerns about benefits. Other concerns which cannot be immediately resolved, such as what, how and when to tell relatives or loved ones about the diagnosis, may be alleviated by drawing up short- and longer-term plans of action with the patient. The overall aim should be to try and help patients achieve a sense of perspective and control regarding their concerns, and not feel they are being ignored or that they are escalating and becoming uncontrollable (Green and McCreaner, 1989).

The following care example also suggests that people with a current mental health problem, particularly if it is acute and unrelated to HIV, may be well advised to wait until they have fully recovered before undertaking a test. A 27-year-old woman with a depressive illness was admitted to an acute ward in a psychiatric hospital. Some years earlier she had shared needles during a relationship with a partner who injected drugs. Although she had no signs of HIV disease and had not expressed any concerns, the registrar suggested an HIV test and the patient had apparently agreed and declined specialist counselling. However, when the result came back positive, the staff were reluctant to tell her because of her already depressed mood. When she was told, she was understandably very distressed and the staff were left feeling that they had added to her mental health concerns rather than caring for her primary reason for being in hospital. This scenario highlights the need to ensure that all clients are helped to consider not only the possible consequences of an HIV antibody test, but also whether this is the best time for them to find out their status.

Previous coping behaviours People tend to repeat previous behaviours in anxiety-provoking situations. If possible, try to get patients to reflect upon how they have coped with similar situations in the past and, if appropriate, relate these coping mechanisms to current concerns. This can also make the problem seem less new and frightening. In addition, it may identify any potentially damaging coping responses, such as substance misuse or self-harm.

Fears about future losses Identify whether the person is worried about possible future losses. The fear of developing dementia-type symptoms may be particularly great, as this quote from a person with AIDS indicates: 'I would rather die from some physical manifestation of AIDS than a neurological one. I would rather die from pneumonia or cancer than lose my grip on reality first and become a non-person even before I am dead' (Masterton and Mordaunt, 1989).

Sometimes the provision of accurate information is reassuring, as it can dispel fears based on misinformation about the prevalence or nature of conditions such as HIV-associated dementia. It is also important to try to assist individuals to explore what it is that they find most frightening about their concerns. For instance, it is often the fear of dying and what this will be like that is more frightening than the idea of death itself. Concerns may be alleviated by talking through how they will be cared for, making it clear that they will be assisted to maintain their dignity and self-respect, with their wishes being respected wherever possible. Assistance to write a treatment plan or an advanced directive may also be welcomed (Schlyter, 1992).

Social support People who feel they have few social supports are at increased risk of psychological distress, and so it is crucial to assess what is available to them at home and in their social circle. They may benefit from engaging with whatever statutory and voluntary services are available and appropriate to their needs. This could include support groups or individual counselling, which may be aimed at particular needs such as those of women, injecting drug users or people from ethnic minorities. Depending on local provision, it may also be possible to offer practical assistance with tasks and responsibilities such as child care, shopping, cooking and decorating.

Many mental health interventions can be carried out by a nurse without any formal mental health training, but if individual nurses feel they are getting out of their depth or do not know how to respond to a concern, they should not hesitate to request advice and assistance from appropriate specialist colleagues, such as a psychiatric nurse, psychologist or psychiatrist.

Psychiatric nurses possess many skills which they can utilize to meet the psychosocial needs of people affected by HIV, provided they have kept themselves up to date with developments in the field of HIV and AIDS. There is clearly a great need for more liaison and community psychiatric nurses to become involved in this area of care, as they are frequently absent from HIV care teams (Grant 1988; Firn, 1992). Their skills include:

- conducting psychiatric nursing assessments which may help clarify problems and identify appropriate nursing interventions;
- providing bereavement and loss therapy;
- identifying problem-solving techniques and promoting effective coping strategies;
- providing education, advice and support to other colleagues in the HIV team.

Psychiatric nurses can also offer to teach anxiety and stress management techniques which may alleviate distress; there have been claims that such interventions can also boost the immune system. These are discussed by King (1993), who concludes that, while there is no clear evidence to support these assertions, they may do much to increase a person's sense of coping and wellbeing, as long as they do not forgo other treatments whose efficacy has been established.

CHANGES IN BODY IMAGE

The devastating changes in body image which can result from some HIV-related illnesses can also have a dramatic effect on a person's psychological wellbeing. The following statement was made by a woman who was interviewed within the framework of a study into the emotional and psychological needs of people with AIDS (Firn and Norman, 1995). She had just been admitted to an inpatient unit for the first time and seen other people with AIDS who had experienced marked weight loss: 'God, was I in a state and everything! Not when I first heard about being positive because I knew there was something wrong. But I didn't realize what a terrible illness it is. I mean, they look like something out of Belsen.' This woman's distress was heightened because she was admitted at night, and said that nobody came to explain to her why she was in hospital or what would happen to her. She said that she discharged herself the next day and took an overdose of analgesics when she returned home. It is crucial that nurses are aware of the potential for such concerns and make every effort to allow patients to ask questions, vent their fears and, if appropriate, get the earliest possible opportunity to speak to a trained counsellor or mental health professional.

Price (1990) described an assessment tool which identifies body reality, body ideal and body presentation as three aspects of body image which, if affected, can lead to psychological trauma. Although not developed specifically for assessing the needs of people with HIV and AIDS, it could be easily adapted to this area of care.

Body reality refers to the actual areas of the body that are affected or likely to be affected. Price maintains that permanent bodily changes, and those affecting the face, hands and sexual organs, are the most significant. These are frequently affected in HIV disease by dramatic weight loss, the disfiguration caused by Kaposi's sarcoma lesions, and repeated infections of the genital areas, such as herpes and thrush. Wherever possible, prevention of such changes should be the primary nursing aim, and this may involve practical interventions such as enabling adequate nutritional intake. If prevention is not possible, efforts can be made to conceal any changes, such as the use of camouflage make-up to cover Kaposi's sarcoma lesions.

Body ideal refers to the individual's internalized personal norms of how they expect their body to appear and function. As previously noted, people affected by HIV tend to be relatively young. Those with high ideals as to their body appearance and function will find it particularly difficult to adapt to changes due to HIV disease. Helping people to alter their expectations and beliefs about their own body is a difficult task which takes time. It may be helpful to consider what it is that the client so cherishes about a particular body ideal, and what it is they will grieve for when it is gone. Price suggests that it can be useful to help patients put changes into context by considering how their body ideal has changed throughout their life, and to try to develop positive ideas about their changed image. The overall goal is to help patients accept their body image and maintain their self-esteem by recognizing that they are still the same person behind their changed appearance and functioning.

Finally, Price cites body presentation as relating to the way a person's body appears to the outside world, e.g. whether they appear ungainly, dexterous or clumsy. Once again, people affected by HIV may experience dramatic changes in this aspect of body image if their central and peripheral nervous system becomes impaired. This can lead to a decline in motor functioning and distressing symptoms such as incontinence. Nursing interventions should focus upon practical interventions which can minimize the effects of these impairments, such as aids and adaptations for eating and mobilizing, along with psychological support aimed at helping the person to feel confident enough to use these in public if necessary.

Sometimes, being sensitive to a person's feelings and acting in an empathic manner when they are distressed about some aspect of body image is all that can be offered, but this can still be extremely therapeutic. In the study previously referred to (Firn and Norman,

1995), patients were asked to identify examples of optimal nursing care one recalled his initial feelings of humiliation after being incontinent, but when the nurse came and sat on the bed and held him and shared his tears, he felt an immense relief and a realization that the nurse cared about him as an individual. He identified this as the best example of a nurse caring for his emotional and psychological needs while in hospital.

NEUROPSYCHIATRIC ASPECTS OF HIV INFECTION

A wide range of neuropsychiatric problems may arise as a result of HIV infection. Some of these are secondary to the complications that follow immunosuppression, and include opportunistic infections affecting the brain, such as toxoplasmosis and cytomegalovirus; tumours such as non-Hodgkin's lymphoma; and concurrent systemic illnesses such as vascular or nutritional disorders, which can also affect cognitive functioning (Everall and Lantos, 1991).

HIV is also known to directly affect the central nervous system (CNS), by crossing the blood–brain barrier within a few weeks of infection. This primary infection of the CNS is responsible for HIV-associated dementia, which can occur in the advanced stages of HIV disease. The exact mechanism by which the virus causes the dementia is unknown. Although up to 90% of people who die of AIDS-related illness have abnormalities in the brain which can be identified at postmortem, only a minority experience clinical symptoms of dementia (Everall and Lantos, 1991). The World Health Organization has suggested that between 8 and 16% of people in the late stages of AIDS will develop HIV-associated dementia, with between 0 and 3.3% doing so as their sole AIDS-defining condition (Maj, 1990b). Thus, severe immunosuppression is almost always necessary before dementia can develop.

Minor symptoms of cognitive and motor impairment do affect a substantial number of people with symptomatic HIV disease (Burgess and Riccio, 1992). A person with minor cognitive impairment may complain of decreased ability to concentrate, forgetfulness and slowed mental functioning. Such patients may, for instance, report difficulties in getting through as much work as they used to, and making mistakes they would not have made in the past. They may also report changes in motor functioning, such as the development of a tremor, loss of feeling in extremities and deteriorating handwriting. However, problems with motor and cognitive functioning do not necessarily occur together and can be mutually exclusive. It is crucial to note that most people with minor cognitive or motor disorder will not develop a clinical dementia.

The essential feature of dementia is a loss of intellectual abilities of sufficient severity to interfere with social or occupational functioning. Affected individuals are likely to have very poor recent memory and experience great difficulties in processing new information. Although they may be lucid and rational at times, at other times they are disorientated regarding time, place and even person. People with HIV-associated dementia tend to become withdrawn and uncommunicative, although they may be more disinhibited in some aspects of their behaviour as previous social norms are disregarded. A person's mood may fluctuate rapidly and irritability is a common feature. Premorbid personality traits are likely to be accentuated. Motor functioning may be further affected, as evidenced by incontinence and impaired mobility (American Academy of Neurology AIDS Task Force, 1991). HIV-associated dementia has to be a diagnosis of exclusion, as it is only by eliminating other possible causes of a person's impaired cognitive or motor functioning, such as the secondary effects of immunosuppression previously described, that a diagnosis of dementia can be made.

It is also important to note that many of the early symptoms of dementia mimic a depressive illness; several studies have shown that, when people with AIDS have been worried about developing dementia, the decrease in their functioning was due to excessive worrying about their health (King, 1993).

ASSESSMENT OF MINOR COGNITIVE AND/OR MOTOR IMPAIRMENT

A full nursing assessment is therefore essential to help clarify the diagnosis, inform nursing care planning and act as a baseline for evaluating later changes. This assessment will complement other investigations, such as EEG, CT and MRI scans and psychometric testing. The assessment should include the following observations, but may need to be adapted depending upon the person's mood and willingness or ability to participate in the assessment (Thomas, 1989; McArthur, 1990):

- Ask the person to give an account of exactly what difficulties he or she has been experiencing, and whether these are really different from the way they usually function. For instance, those worried about developing dementia may not recognize how they used to forget appointments before their diagnosis. If possible, get an account from another person who knows the patient well, such as a partner or work colleague.

- Carry out a simple mental state test by checking the person's short-term memory, orientation and knowledge of current events. Observe level of attention and concentration, whether they are able to follow your conversation, and the content of their speech. Note personal appearance, and determine whether it seems in keeping with background.
- Assess any evidence of nervous system impairment by observing whether the person has any slurring of speech, weakness in limbs, or problems with fine movement or general mobility.
- Assess whether the person is excessively anxious or is ruminating about his or her health. This should include questions about concentration levels, the existence of recurring negative thoughts, and the degree of awareness of bodily responses. For instance, has he or she experienced sweating, palpitations or feelings of panic?
- Explore whether the person is experiencing any psychological stresses or has suffered any recent losses. These can precipitate minor declines in cognitive functioning, and the person may find it reassuring to know that people living with other life-threatening conditions have also been shown to function less well.
- Assess whether the person has a history or current symptoms of depressive illness. Traditional markers such as decreased appetite, weight loss and disturbed sleep pattern are not reliable indicators because many people with HIV experience these changes irrespective of their mood. Focus should be on the person's self-image and self-esteem. This includes examining whether levels of interest in everyday activities and social contact are maintained. Check whether the person views him- or herself as being just as likeable and successful as in the past, and if he or she is looking forward to anything in the future. It is also vital to check whether there are any mood fluctuations at different times of the day, and if there have been any thoughts about suicide or self-harm (Swanson et al., 1990).
- Assess whether the person has engaged in excessive alcohol consumption or used non-prescribed drugs.
- Check whether the person has any concurrent physical illness, or if any medication is being taken which may affect functioning.

If in any doubt, nurses should refer to a specialist colleague such as a psychiatrist, psychologist or neurologist. However, there are no psychometric tests or other investigations capable of predicting who will progress from comparatively minor impairment to dementia.

CARE OF PEOPLE WITH HIV-ASSOCIATED DEMENTIA

With patients who have developed dementia, the nurse's main role is to enable and empower them to maintain a sense of control and dignity and to optimize their quality of life in accordance with their care preferences.

The most important concern is safety. Short-term memory loss, disorientation, poor concentration and decreased awareness of danger may all contribute to risks such as fire from cooking or discarded cigarettes, wandering at night, or accidental overdose with medication. Periods of lucidity and insight may precipitate self-harm. Motor impairment may cause falls or burns. Each one of these risks should be assessed within the context of the person's degree of impairment, environment and level of support.

Practical steps can be taken to minimize the risk of self-harm by ensuring the environment is as safe as possible. This may include, for instance, preventing falls by making sure that there are no electrical leads that could trip up the patient, as well as liaising with an occupational therapist and social worker in order to provide aids and equipment such as a walking stick, handrails and adapted cups and utensils. Medication can be provided in boxes, with each dose in a separate compartment, enabling the person to check whether medication has been taken at the due time and minimize the risk of accidental overdose.

Other coping strategies can be drawn from interventions developed in the care of the elderly, such as helping the person establish the practice of consulting a prominently displayed calendar upon which a carer has written all appointments and visitors. A structured and consistent routine is essential for a person with dementia, and so care should be planned around the minimum number of people necessary to meet the person's needs, who should attempt to call at the same time whenever possible. Even if the person is unable to remember somebody's name or occupation, he or she is very likely to recognize the face of a frequent visitor and this is the basis for a trusting and therapeutic relationship.

Communication is at the heart of providing care in this area (Bartol, 1979). Table 13.1 provides a list of suggestions for enabling communication with a person with cognitive impairment.

If a person still retains periods of lucidity and insight, it may be possible to help him or her plan ahead and attend to unfinished business. This may include saying goodbye to loved ones, or indicating preferences regarding care by making a treatment plan, thereby helping the person maintain a sense of dignity and control and easing fears about not being able to communicate in the future.

Table 13.1 Sensitive communication with a person with severe cognitive impairment

- Allow plenty of time for the conversation.
- Begin each conversation by introducing yourself and calling the person by his or her name.
- Be aware of your non-verbal communication. If possible, sit down and try to look open and relaxed.
- Try not to make sudden movements.
- Speak slowly and say individual words clearly.
- Repeat yourself if necessary. Never raise your voice unless the person cannot hear what you are saying.
- Ask one question at a time, avoiding lengthy sentences containing a number of points or questions.
- Allow the person plenty of time to reply.
- Tell the person if you do not understand what he or she is saying and ask him or her to repeat.
- Maintain eye contact.
- Check for understanding by reflecting back statements and summarizing issues. Ask the person to repeat back key points.
- Look out for specific interventions that seem to work for particular situations. Ask partners and significant others for advice.
- If you say you are going to do something for the person, do it. Do not assume it will be forgotten. If you are unable to do something, or forget, explain the reason to the person.
- If the person becomes angry or threatening, it may be necessary to end the conversation. However, try to find out what precipitated the reaction, perhaps by going back a few minutes later and asking.

It can be extremely distressing for loved ones to watch someone lose their cognitive abilities, and they may find themselves saying goodbye well before that person's death, leading to anticipatory grief. Informal carers and partners may then need assistance to work through the grief process. This can be carried out on an individual basis or through support groups. The latter are often helpful if the partner is also infected, or feels guilty about having transmitted the virus to the loved one (Flaskerud, 1992). Lasher and Ragsdale (1989) outline ways in which significant others can participate in the planning and provision of care, which may help to ease their sense of loss and helplessness. Providing 24-hour care for someone with HIV-associated dementia can be extremely stressful and exhausting, and informal carers should be given information and assistance in obtaining help, which may relieve some of the pressure. This could include day care, respite care, night sitting and practical help with chores such as shopping and cooking.

People with HIV-associated dementia often require hospitalization, either because of concurrent physical illness, safety needs or because no one is able to manage their care at home. When this is the case, it is preferable that people are cared for in a general hospital ward to facilitate optimum treatment of their systemic illnesses and minimize distress. This seems extremely difficult to achieve in a psychiatric setting. Acute psychiatric wards are often very noisy, busy and distressing to people with dementia, especially young people, who would be cared for among elderly people with mental illness. However, general nurses caring for people with HIV-associated dementia should be supported by psychiatric nursing colleagues visiting the ward and providing whatever advice, support, education and interventions are required to ensure that the client's mental health needs are met. This may involve an educative role, explaining the possible reasons for any seemingly bizarre or threatening behaviour exhibited by the patient, and responding to any questions, fears or concerns expressed by the nurses. It may also involve advising on interventions and planning care based on a comprehensive, thorough assessment (Grant, 1988).

Occasionally admission to psychiatric hospital is necessary, particularly if the person has acute behavioural disturbances and cannot be safely cared for in any other setting. However, we were recently told by a nurse managing a psychiatric ward that they could not admit a person with AIDS, even though he was physically well, because the staff did not have the requisite knowledge or skills and she 'needed a few days to prepare them'. Such statements are entirely unacceptable, as the UKCC (1992) have made clear that every nurse has a duty to maintain up-to-date professional knowledge and competence. Baer *et al.* (1987) describe the experience of caring for people with HIV-associated dementia in a psychiatric ward in the United States. They point out that, in addition to the need to educate staff, there was a need to educate other patients who became aware of or guessed the patient's diagnosis. Such patients expressed fears of 'catching AIDS', had difficulty in believing that young people could suffer from dementia and accused them of receiving special treatment, and a few incorporated issues around AIDS into their delusions.

PSYCHOSES IN PEOPLE WITH HIV DISEASE

It has been widely noted in the literature that a minority of people with HIV infection may experience psychotic illnesses, which are characterized by a lack of insight into their illness and a loss of contact with some aspects of reality. The most commonly occurring disorders are affective disorders, such as severe depression and mania, and schizophrenic-type illnesses (Catalan, 1993). The aetiology of such conditions is unknown, and a debate is continuing as to whether there is an 'HIV-specific psychosis' (Vogel-Scibilia *et al.*, 1988; Maj, 1990a), that is, whether a psychotic illness may occur which is due to the effects of HIV acting on the nervous system, or whether their occurrence is coincidental. A further postulation is that some people may have a predisposition to such illness which is exacerbated by the stress of diagnosis (Richardson, 1992).

King (1993) points out that mania appears to predominate among the psychotic illnesses affecting people with HIV. He further states that these are often atypical forms of mania, in that the person is more irritable than euphoric and may not fully recover their previous judgement. This suggests that a degree of cognitive impairment may have occurred. He cautiously concludes that in such cases there may be some unidentified organic pathology, particularly if there is no personal or family history of similar disorders.

What is clear is that psychotic illnesses most commonly occur in the late stages of HIV disease. This means that a person will frequently have concurrent physical conditions, which in turn implies that, once again, psychiatric nurses will need to work closely with general nursing colleagues to provide holistic care.

SUMMARY

It is clearly established that a wide range of mental health problems are related to HIV infection and AIDS, and that these may occur throughout the HIV disease process. Because of the dynamic nature of the condition people frequently experience a multiplicity of problems, creating concurrent physical, social and mental health needs. Thus, all nurses involved in the care of people affected by HIV need to incorporate a basic understanding of mental health concerns into their assessments, as well as being aware of the types of interventions that may be beneficial, and knowing how to contact other specialist agencies.

Some people who are not infected become chronically anxious about acquiring HIV, or over-concerned that they have already been infected (Miller *et al.*, 1988; Davey and Green, 1991). Whenever individuals with these concerns are not reassured by factual information, counselling and negative HIV antibody tests, they should be offered referral to a mental health professional as there is frequently an underlying cause which is not directly related to HIV. Nursing assessments of such concerns have been outlined (Flaskerud, 1992) and nursing interventions have been suggested (Mathews, 1988).

Psychosocial reactions to infection most commonly occur at times of change and loss, and include adjustment disorders, anxiety disorders and mood disturbances. The periods when people are most vulnerable appear to be following an HIV or AIDS diagnosis, when physical symptoms emerge, and when treatment or prophylaxis commences. People with few social supports and those with a history of a previous psychiatric illness seem most at risk of developing a mental health problem, along with those who inject drugs (Catalan, 1993). All nursing assessments should be informed by this knowledge, and should help to determine at which stages of the HIV disease process it is important to focus resources in response to patients' needs at that time. Psychiatric nurses are able to provide a number of interventions which may be beneficial, including bereavement and loss therapy, problem-solving techniques, and the promotion of coping strategies (Korniewicz *et al.*, 1990; Firn, 1992).

A number of neuropsychiatric conditions have been identified, although these rarely occur in the absence of severe immuno-suppression, the complications of which can lead to opportunistic infections, tumours and other systemic illnesses that affect the functioning of the nervous system. Primary infection of the nervous system by HIV is associated with the development of a clinical dementia. This can have devastating effects on cognitive and motor functioning and cause severe behavioural disturbance, but is thankfully much less common than was feared a few years ago (Everall and Lantos, 1991). A number of potentially treatable conditions can present similar symptoms to early-stage dementia, including depression, and nurses have a crucial role in assessing for differential diagnoses (McArthur, 1990). The main role of the nurse in the care of someone with HIV-associated dementia is to maintain safety while striving to promote control, dignity and independence. Many of the skills developed in the care of the elderly mentally ill may be adapted to this area of care, although it is not appropriate to use elderly care services. The changes brought about by HIV-associated dementia can be particularly distressing for partners, relatives and significant others, and their needs must also be addressed (Lasher and Ragsdale, 1989).

A small number of people develop severe psychiatric illnesses, such as hypomania and major depression, but the role and significance of HIV in the development of such conditions is unknown (Maj, 1990a). Nevertheless, people with such conditions often require admission to psychiatric hospital, and this emphasizes the need for all psychiatric nurses to maintain an adequate knowledge base around HIV and to demonstrate the qualities of self-awareness and non-judgemental attitudes for which the profession often claims praise.

The dynamic nature of HIV disease also demands a holistic approach to care and the development of close liaisons and shared expertise between general and psychiatric nursing colleagues and other members of the HIV care team. This includes those working in non-statutory organizations, who frequently take the lead in providing emotional and psychological support.

REFERENCES

Aggleton, P. and Homans, H. (eds) (1988) *Social Aspects of AIDS*, Falmer Press, Lewes.

American Academy of AIDS Neurology Taskforce (1991) Nomenclature and research case definitions for neurological manifestations of human immunodeficiency virus type-1 (HIV-1) infections. *Neurology*, **41**, 778–85.

Asher, R. (1951) Munchausen's syndrome. *Lancet*, **i**, 3339–41.

Baer, J.W., Hall, J.M. and Holm, K. (1987) Challenges in developing an in-patient psychiatric program for patients with AIDS and ARC. *Hospital and Community Psychiatry*, **38**, 1299–303.

Bartol, M.A. (1979) Non-verbal communication in patients with Alzheimer's disease. *Journal of Gerontological Nursing*, **5**, 21.

Burgess, A. and Riccio, M. (1992) Cognitive impairment and dementia in HIV-1 infection. *Baillière's Clinical Neurology*, **1**, 155–74.

Burnard, P. (1993) The psychosocial needs of people with HIV and AIDS: a view from nurse educators and counsellors. *Journal of Advanced Nursing*, **18**, 1779–86.

Catalan, J. (1993) *HIV Infection and Mental Health Care: Implications for Services*, World Health Organization Regional Office for Europe, Second report, WHO, Geneva.

Davey, T. and Green, J. (1991) The worried well: ten years of a new face for an old problem. *AIDS Care*, **3**(3), 289–93.

Everall, I.P. and Lantos, P.L. (1991) The neuropathology of HIV: review of the first ten years. *International Review of Psychiatry*, **3**, 307–20.

Firn, S. (1992) Responding to HIV: facing the challenge. *Nursing Times*, **88**(37), 60–2.

Firn, S. and Norman, I. (1995) Psychological and emotional impact of an HIV diagnosis. *Nursing Times*, **91**(8), 37–9.

Flaskerud, J.H. (1992) Psychosocial aspects, in *HIV/AIDS: a guide to nursing care*, 2nd edn, (eds J. H. Flaskerud and P. J. Ungvarski), W.B. Saunders, Philadelphia, pp. 239–74.

Gala, C., Pergami, A., Catalan, J. *et al.* (1993) The psychosocial impact of HIV infection in gay men, drug users and heterosexuals. *British Journal of Psychiatry*, **163**, 651–9.

Grant, S.M. (1988) The hospitalized AIDS patient and the psychiatric liaison nurse. *Archives of Psychiatric Nursing*, **2**(1), 35–9.

Green, J. and McCreaner, A. (1989) *Counselling in HIV Infection and AIDS*, Blackwell Scientific, Oxford.

King, M. (1989) Psychosocial status of 192 outpatients with HIV infection and AIDS. *British Journal of Psychiatry*, **154**, 237–42.

King, M. (1990) Psychological aspects of HIV Infection and AIDS: what have we learned? *British Journal of Psychiatry*, **156**, 151–6.

King, M. (1993) *AIDS, HIV and Mental Health*, Cambridge University Press, Cambridge.

Korniewicz, D.M., O'Brien, M.E. and Larson, E. (1990) Coping with AIDS and HIV. *Journal of Psychosocial Nursing*, **28**(3), 14–21.

Lasher, A.T. and Ragsdale, D. (1989) The significant other's role in improving the quality of life in persons with AIDS dementia complex. *Journal of Neuroscience Nursing*, **21**(4), 250–5.

Lewin, C. and Williams, R.J.W. (1988) Fear of AIDS: the impact of public anxiety in young people. *British Journal of Psychiatry*, **153**, 823–4.

McArthur, J. (1990) AIDS Dementia: your assessment can make all the difference. *RN*, March, 36–42.

McDonald, J. and Wafer, K. (1989) Munchausen syndrome masquerading as AIDS-induced depression. Letter. *British Journal of Psychiatry*, **154**, 420–1.

Maj, M. (1990a) Psychiatric aspects of HIV infection and AIDS. *Psychological Medicine*, **20**, 547–63.

Maj, M. (1990b) Organic mental disorders in HIV-1 infection. *AIDS*, **4**, 831–40.

Masterton, J. and Mordaunt, J. (1989) *Facing up to AIDS*, O'Brien Press, Dublin.

Mathews, S. J. (1988) Nothing to fear but fear. *Nursing Times*, **84**(28), 35–7.

Miller, D. and Riccio, M. (1990) Non-organic psychiatric and psychosocial syndromes associated with HIV-1 infection and disease. *AIDS*, **4**, 381–8.

Miller, D., Acton, T.M.G. and Hedge, B. (1988) The worried well: their identification and management. *Journal of the Royal College of Physicians of London*, **22**(3), 158–65.

Price, B. (1990) *Body Image: Nursing Concepts and Care*, Prentice Hall, Hemel Hempstead.

Richardson, A. (1992) Psychiatric and neuropsychological aspects, in *Reflective Helping in HIV and AIDS*, (eds C. Anderson and P. Wilkie), Open University Press, Milton Keynes.

Schlyter, C. (1992) *Advance Directives and AIDS: an Empirical Study of the Interest in Living Wills and Proxy Decision Making in the Context of HIV/AIDS Care*, Centre of Medical Law and Ethics, King's College, University of London.

Swanson, B., Cronin-Stubbs, D. and Colletti, M.A. (1990) Dementia and depression in persons with AIDS: causes and care. *Journal of Psychosocial Nursing*, **28**(10), 33–9.

Thomas, B. (1989) HIV and encephalopathy. *Nursing*, 3(46), 4–7.

UKCC (1992) *Code of Professional Conduct for the Nurse, Midwife and Health Visitor*, UKCC, London.

Vogel-Scibilia, S.E., Mulsant, B.H. and Keshavan, M.S. (1988) HIV infection presenting as psychosis: a critique. *Acta Psychiatrica Scandinavica*, **78**, 652–6.

Establishing a nursing agenda for HIV/AIDS 14

Ian Hicken and Jean Faugier

A recurrent theme throughout this book has been how nurses have risen to the challenges posed by HIV infection and AIDS. Inevitably, nursing responses have been driven by a range of influences from within health and social care provision, and by pressures exerted by those affected by HIV/AIDS. However, for many nurses HIV/AIDS has served as the catalyst which has brought to the fore many social and political injustices in today's society, which are therefore implicit in health care. Issues such as equity in health care, oppression, discrimination and victim blaming, the taboos of sex and sexuality, drug use and misuse, empowerment and disempowerment, and the fear of contagion have all been integral to the HIV/AIDS debate. Of course these issues are not just related to HIV/AIDS, they have been present in society throughout history. What is different with HIV/AIDS is that for probably the first time in the history of health care, the nursing profession has realized that, with adequate resources in terms of accurate and accessible information and the will to change and influence outcomes, health and social care workers, working together towards a common goal, can affect how things will be. At a very basic level nurses can make a difference; the problems are not insurmountable. Richard Wells, to whom this book is dedicated, once said that 'if we get it right for people with AIDS then we will get it right for everyone else'. His words have been quoted many times and for many nurses they encapsulate feelings which until the emergence of HIV/AIDS had no 'collective voice'.

The 'collective voice' has achieved a great deal over the past decade, but questions need to be asked as to why, despite all the lobbying, HIV/AIDS still brings out the worst in human behaviour and attitudes? Perhaps by making HIV/AIDS the vehicle for change, we only reinforce and strengthen the negative attitudes and feelings of fear and insecurity towards the issues raised. Could it be that for many people HIV/AIDS brings an unacceptable focus to a multitude of issues, which together are too overpowering and overwhelming?

The evolution of HIV and AIDS brought with it a tier of specialist workers without whom many of the innovative practices and treatments would not have been developed. However, in many instances this has reinforced the notion that HIV and AIDS is special. In part, this has been due to the reluctance of some specialist workers to 'let go' and allow their colleagues from generic services to become involved. The reasons for this are complex and potentially controversial. Are the reasons why HIV/AIDS has remained within the specialist arena purely related to the perceived inability of non-specialist workers to adequately care for people with the disease? Surely it is illogical on the one hand to promulgate the belief that HIV/AIDS is everyone's concern, and yet on the other hand make it difficult for everyone to get involved? One reason put forward for continuing the specialist focus of HIV/AIDS work is that those affected do not trust generic services, i.e. they do not have the expertise nor the mechanisms to ensure confidentiality. All nurses are bound by the Code of Professional Conduct, and as such have a duty to care and maintain confidentiality. If nurses refuse to care, or if that care is not adequate, or if confidentiality is broken, then there are clear, unambiguous mechanisms in place to address these issues. How can colleagues working in generic services be expected to gain experience if they are not permitted to care for those affected? Surely we have a duty to promote generic services to patients and reassure them that a quality service will be provided? Funding has been cited as another reason why HIV/AIDS has, in the main, continued to be located within the specialist arena. Many HIV/AIDS-related posts have been established and funded by the availability of earmarked monies. Could it be that by promoting the use of generic services, those who are reliant on such monies for employment would jeopardize their position?

There is an urgent need to examine the role of the specialist worker, to explore how they can support and enable the generic worker to effectively care for people affected by HIV/AIDS. The mainstreaming of HIV/AIDS will require specialist workers to develop their skills of advocacy, not only for people affected by HIV/AIDS but also of generic services and staff, which are more than able to provide quality care but only if they are empowered through information, support and experience.

The Government's move to mainstream HIV/AIDS care and treatment will inevitably mean that earmarked monies are gradually integrated into global budgets. It will become increasingly difficult to secure high levels of funding to maintain existing services, or to justify monies for developing new services. The mainstreaming of HIV/AIDS funding and care provision will require the nursing profession to re-examine its role in HIV/AIDS care. There will be an increased emphasis on demonstrating to purchasers that a nursing contribution to HIV/AIDS care is cost-effective, value for money and justified. Nursing interventions informed by research will need to be clearly identified and demonstrated as to how they complement and enhance the totality of care within a multiprofessional framework. Outcomes which can be measured and qualified will need to be established and evaluated. A priority for nursing in the future will be to contribute much more visibly to the purchaser–provider cycle by clearly identifying its role in the commissioning process and the evaluation of service provision. Nurses are uniquely positioned to contribute to the contracting process by challenging clinical practice, challenging the basis of prices, evaluating alternatives, interpreting users' needs and contributing to quality (NHSME, 1994).

As we enter the new 'market-driven' NHS culture, demand for resources will undoubtedly exceed supply. With a greater emphasis on mainstreaming HIV/AIDS services, greater accountability of HIV/AIDS-related expenditure and a call to find the right balance with other health priorities, nursing has to be prepared to put forward rational justifications for maintaining the impetus of work to date. Stewart (1993) asked 'should AIDS be given priority in expenditure, institutional and community care over heart disease with over 200 000 deaths annually, or cancer with over 100 000 deaths or an ageing population with all of these and more?'

Underpinning the HIV/AIDS debate is the fact that the virus has the potential to infiltrate all sections of society, and as such the cost is potentially devastating. All health and social care workers have a responsibility to maximize their efforts to eradicate the further spread of HIV by actively promoting the sexual health of the nation. All nurses are in a position to influence the health and wellbeing of patients and clients with whom they come into contact. However, without commitment and support from management, nurses will continue to find it difficult to secure the education and training they may need to adequately fulfil this role. Over the past few years there have been several initiatives that aim to prepare nurses, midwives and health visitors for their role in HIV and sexual health-related practice (ENB, 1994). Not least of these is the move by the ENB to ensure that appropriate attention is given to sexual health within preregistration education and training programmes. Guidelines on how sexual health can be integrated into all nursing curricula have been developed (Hicken, 1994) and widely circulated. The rationale for this work is based on the belief that until nurses are educated and prepared for their role in the wider context of sexual health, and all that sexual health embraces, then they will not be in a position to care effectively for people who present with specific sexually related diseases, such as HIV infection. Similarly, the ENB has recently commenced a project on substance misuse education and training in an attempt to identify and address the deficits in current education and training programmes. Although these initiatives are welcomed, it is crucial that ongoing monitoring of nurse education takes place to ensure that these issues are not subsumed by other pressing educational issues, which may be determined by local demand.

Dialogue between providers and purchasers of nurse education must continue to address issues such as HIV, sexual health and drug use within the context of mainstream nurse education and training. All nurses must be able to recognize the impact of these issues on health and wellbeing, and have a working knowledge of where specialist support and advice can be obtained.

Lack of knowledge and inappropriate attitudes towards HIV/AIDS and related issues among health-care workers has been well documented and referenced within this book. Education and training, access to information and support from the specialist workers without doubt help to overcome some of the difficulties nurses have experienced when faced with the prospect of caring for someone affected by HIV/AIDS. However, in the main HIV/AIDS is not the problem. Closer examination of the research on nurses' knowledge and attitudes towards HIV/AIDS suggests that issues such as lifestyle, sexuality and discrimination override the fear of contagion. Obviously these are not issues which are solely linked to HIV/AIDS. Lack of understanding about different lifestyles, discrimination in its many forms and the taboo of sexuality are inherent in British society, and are reflected in some health-care systems. There are many social issues which still challenge us as nurses, including sex and sexuality; access and equity in health care for a range of client groups; drug use; race and ethnicity; culture and religion. We have learnt a great deal from HIV/AIDS and its impact on individuals, institutions and society alike. The time has come to extrapolate our new-found knowledge and awareness to health and wellbeing, health and social care, and the role and responsibilities of the nursing profession. The words of Richard Wells in the mid-1980s gave us a collective voice and an ideal which served as a benchmark for nursing and HIV/AIDS at a time when passions were high and the motivation to change the way things were was high on the nursing agenda. These lessons from the nursing response to HIV/AIDS, both positive and negative, combined with the experience of those living with the disease, has helped us to make many advances in care. We now need to resist focusing solely on HIV/AIDS and utilize our collective vision to get it right for everyone; only then will we be able to get it right for people affected by HIV/AIDS.

REFERENCES

ENB (1994) *Final Report of the HIV/AIDS Education and Training Project 1990–1994*, ENB, London.

Hicken, I. (1994) *Sexual Health Education and Training: Guidelines for Good Practice in the Teaching of Nurses, Midwives and Health Visitors*, ENB, London.

NHSME (1994) *Building a Stronger Team: The Nursing Contribution to Purchasing. A Report*, NHSME, Leeds.

Stewart, G. (1993) Predictable and preventable? *Nursing Times*, **89**(26), 29–32.

Index